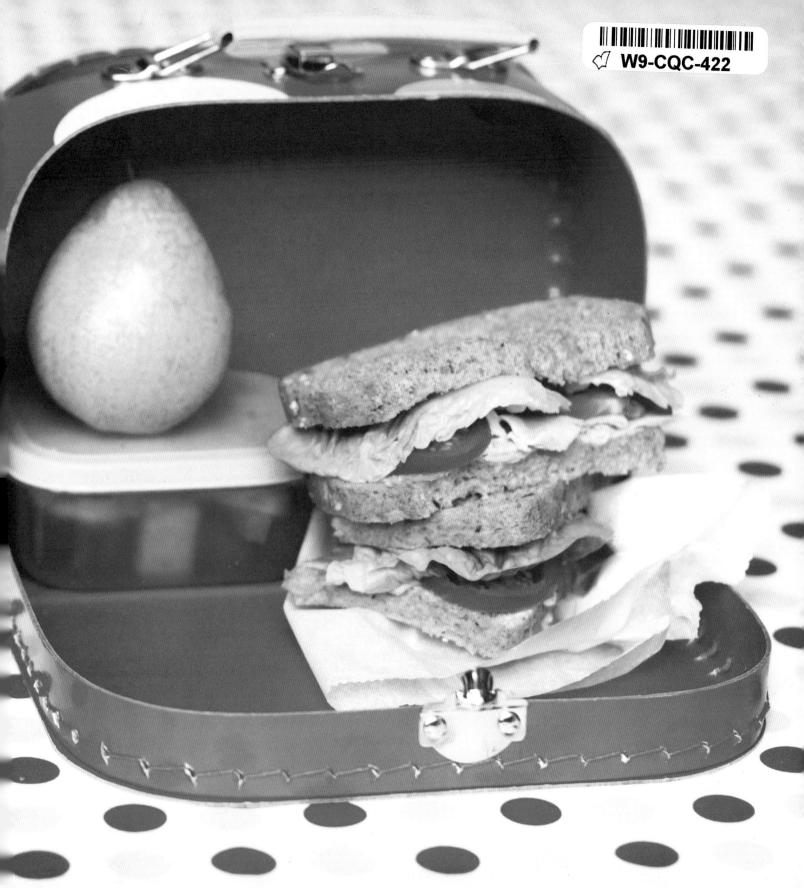

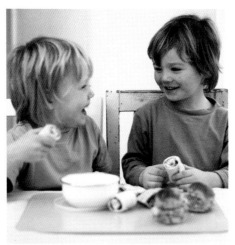

# healthy lunchboxes
*for kids*

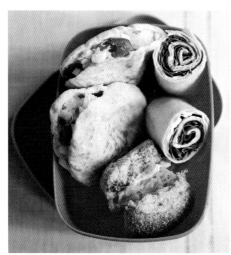

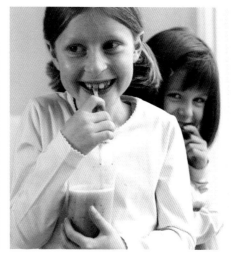

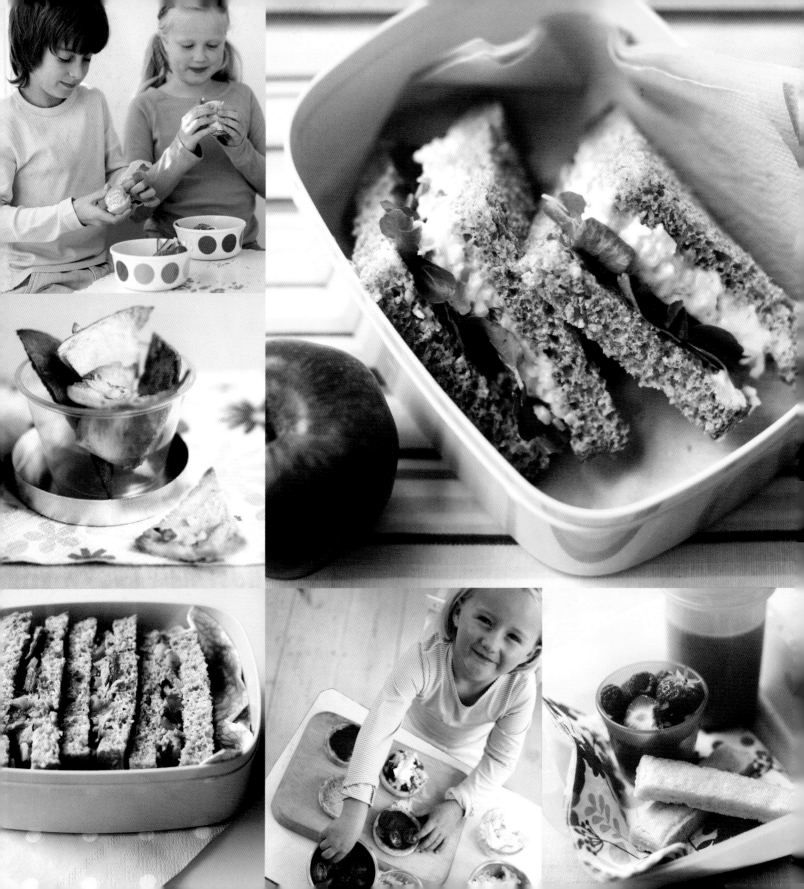

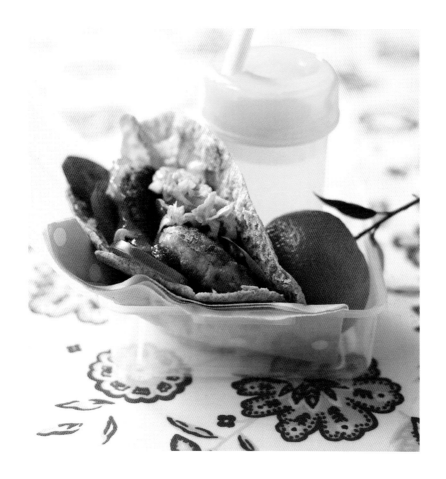

# healthy lunchboxes
## *for kids*

### Amanda Grant

*photography by* Tara Fisher

RYLAND
PETERS
& SMALL
LONDON NEW YORK

**Designer** Iona Hoyle
**Senior Editor** Catherine Osborne
**Production Manager** Patricia Harrington
**Art Director** Leslie Harrington
**Publishing Director** Alison Starling

**Food Stylists** Amanda Grant and Jacque Malouf
**Prop Stylist** Liz Belton
**Indexer** Ann Barrett

First published in the United States in 2008
by Ryland Peters & Small, inc.
519 Broadway, 5th Floor
New York NY10012
www.rylandpeters.com

10 9 8 7 6 5 4 3 2

Text, design, and photographs
© 2008 Ryland Peters & Small

Library of Congress Cataloging-in-Publication Data

Grant, Amanda.
  Healthy lunchboxes for kids / Amanda Grant ;
photography by Tara Fisher.
-- 1st American ed.
    p. cm.
  Includes index.
  ISBN 978-1-84597-706-1 (pbk. : alk. paper)
  1. Lunchbox cookery. 2. Children--Nutrition. I.
Title.
  TX735.G68 2008
  641.5'3--dc22
                        2008023497

ISBN: 978 1 84597 706 1

Printed in China

**Notes**

▪ All spoon measurements are level
unless otherwise specified.
▪ Ovens should be preheated to the specified
temperatures. All ovens work slightly differently.
We recommend using an oven thermometer and
suggest you consult the maker's handbook for any
special instructions, particularly if you are cooking
in a fan-assisted oven, as you will need to adjust
temperatures according to manufacturer's
instructions.
▪ All eggs are medium, unless otherwise specified.
Recipes containing raw or partially cooked egg, or
raw fish or shellfish, should not be served to the
very young, very old, anyone with a compromised
immune system or pregnant women. It is
recommended that free-range eggs be used
throughout.

Neither the author nor the publisher can be held
responsible for any claim arising out of the
information in this book. Always consult your
health advisor or doctor if you have any concerns
about your child's health or nutrition.

# contents

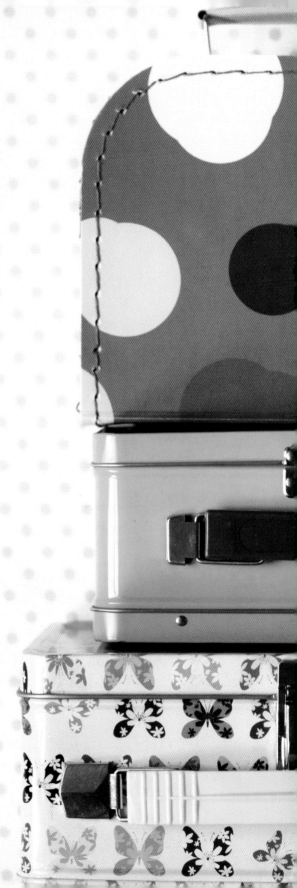

6   introduction

14   the perfect lunchbox

16   sandwiches

38   one-pot salads

52   hot food

64   savories

86   snacks

100   something sweet

122   packaging

124   menu planner

126   index

128   acknowledgments

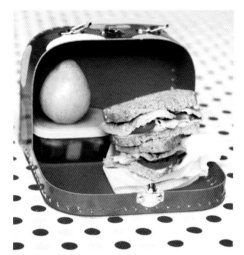

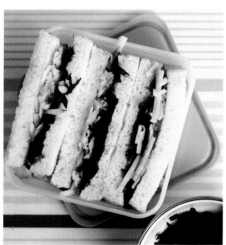

# introduction

### the perfect lunchbox

What foods should you pack into your child's lunchbox? If you're a busy parent, it can be challenging to come up with options that are nutritious, practical and affordable, and, most importantly, that children enjoy eating.

Millions of children take a bag lunch or lunchbox to school every weekday. Surveys have shown that those who eat a hot school lunch are more likely to have a balanced healthy meal than those who "brown bag" it. Many bag or box lunches contain foods too high in saturated fat, salt or sugar, such as potato chips, candy, cookies, sugary drinks, sodas and other highly processed snacks.

A diet that is high in fat, salt and refined carbohydrates not only lays the foundations for heart disease and high blood pressure later in life, but can also contribute to reduced mental alertness, tiredness and lack of concentration in school.

Despite what many manufacturers promote, highly processed foods that are packaged in brightly coloured plastic are not what we should be giving our children. The food is often poor quality, and you are mostly paying for the elaborate packaging and advertising.

Instead, you can save money and give children a better start in life by providing them with good nutritious food. With some forethought and a little time, you can make a healthy lunchbox of fresh and unprocessed food—the sort of food that our parents grew up eating before manufacturers tapped into the children's snack market. Next time you have a roast chicken or roast beef for example, save some cold meat to put in lunchbox sandwiches the next day.

Try to think of providing bag lunches as the perfect opportunity for setting some basic principles about eating good food, rather than seeing it as a chore. Lunch should provide children with approximately one third of their daily energy needs as well as one third of their required protein, carbohydrate, vitamin, mineral and fiber intake. Refer to page 14 for an example of the perfect healthy lunchbox, and use this as your guide to preparing achievable lunches each day. If you can feed your children a healthy diet 80 per cent of the time, then you are doing pretty well.

### the perfect lunchbox

A perfect lunchbox should contain (see page 14 for further information):

- 1 serving of a protein-rich food
- 1 serving of carbohydrate or starchy food
- 1 serving of a calcium-rich food
- 1 serving of fruit
- 1 serving of vegetables
- 1 drink

## "fast"-food basics

Before you start reading about how to make a healthy lunchbox, don't forget that children need a nutritious breakfast before they go to school. This meal needs to provide them with enough energy to get them through the morning. High-sugar breakfasts, like cereals coated in sugar, are best avoided because they will only provide short-lived energy. Instead, start the day with oatmeal made with low-fat milk, granola or muesli with 1% or skim milk, or wholewheat toast with some scrambled egg or peanut butter.

Continue on the right path by packing some healthy mid-morning snacks in your child's lunchbox that provide slow-release energy, like fresh fruit or vegetables, cereal bars or rice cakes with dip (see pages 92–93). To help keep your child's mood and behaviour on an even keel, and to help him/her concentrate in class during the afternoon, make sure you provide a nutritionally balanced lunchbox.

The *My Pyramid Healthy Eating Guide* (available at MyPyramid.gov) will help guide you in making healthy food choices

## protein foods

Foods high in protein include meat, chicken, fish, eggs, beans, lentils, and nuts. These foods are vital for our child's growth and brain development. A popular myth is that the more protein you give children, the quicker they will grow and develop, but this isn't the case. Protein is made up of building blocks called amino acids, of which there are 22. Most of these can be made in our body from proteins except for an essential 8 (or 9 in children) that must come from our food.

Protein is either animal-based or vegetable-based. Animal proteins, such as chicken, fish, meat, and eggs contain all the essential amino acids. Plant proteins are referred to as incomplete proteins because they don't contain all of the essential amino acids. If you wish to feed your child a vegetarian diet, you will need to make sure that it is a combination of grains, nuts, seeds, pulses and beans to give a complete balance of these essential amino acids. Protein-rich foods are also good sources of some B vitamins, iron, and zinc.

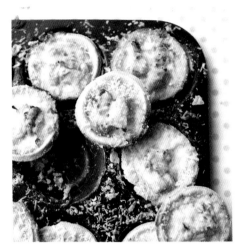

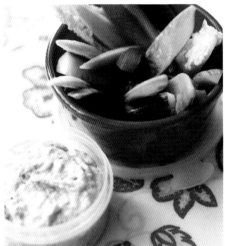

### *protein requirement*

Every packed lunch should contain 1 serving of food from the meat, poultry, fish, dry beans, eggs, and nuts group. As a rule, children need 2–3 servings of these foods each day.

For children aged 5–8 years, a serving is:
- 1½ oz. sliced lean cooked meat or poultry
- 1–2 tablespoons peanut butter
- 1½ oz. fish
- 1 egg
- ½ cup cooked beans

For children aged 9–11 years, a serving is:
- 2–3 oz. sliced lean meat or poultry
- 2–3 tablespoons peanut butter
- 2–3 oz. fish
- 1–2 eggs
- ½–1 cup cooked beans

\*Note: For fish and egg recipes see pages 32, 35, 40, 43, 80–82.

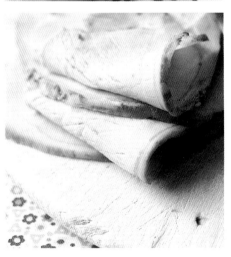

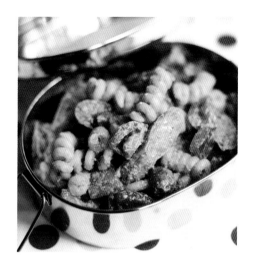

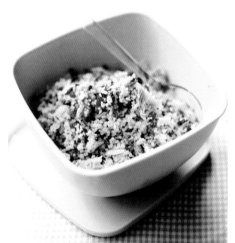

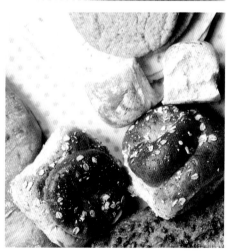

## carbohydrate foods

These provide a steady stream of energy and help keep sugar levels balanced. They are typically found in unrefined and whole-grain foods, which are richer in nutrients and fiber than their refined equivalents. Good slow-release carbohydrates include oats, wholewheat breads, and baked products made with whole-grains, brown rice, and wholewheat pasta .

### carbohydrate requirement

Every packed lunch should contain 1 or more servings of foods from the bread, potatoes, and other cereals group (depending on how much is provided in other meals). As a rule, children need at least 6 servings a day.

For children aged 5–8 years, a serving may be:
- 1 small slice bread
- ½ small roll
- ½–¾ cup pasta or rice
- ½–¾ cup dry breakfast cereal

For children aged 9–11 years, a serving may be:
- 1 slice bread
- ½–1 small roll
- ½–¾ cup pasta or rice
- ¾–1 cup dry breakfast cereal

*Note: For potato, pasta and cereal recipes see pages 42–45 and 120.

Fast-releasing carbohydrates, on the other hand, include high-sugar foods made with lots of unrefined sugar, like cookies and cakes, and baked goods that contain high fat and white flour, like croissants and muffins.

It is fine to include some fast-releasing carbohydrates in your child's diet, but to help slow down the rate at which they rush through the bloodstream, it is a good idea to combine them with protein-rich food. For example, white rice is best served with chicken or fish. This is simply because proteins take a longer time to digest and hence slow down the absorption of the fast-releasing sugars.

As a general guide, children over the age of 5 years should be eating two thirds whole-grain foods, like wholewheat pasta and wholewheat bread, and one third white flour products, such as pasta, rice, etc. Make sure you include slow-release carbohydrates in your child's diet.

## fiber

If you increase the number of slow-release carbohydrates in your child's diet, you will also increase their fiber intake. Fiber is important for a number of reasons—it maintains the health of the digestive tract, slows down the release of sugars into the bloodstream, helps the body eliminate toxins, and feeds beneficial bacteria that are found in the gut.

If children are fed a processed diet that is high in refined foods, and hence less fiber, they are more likely to suffer from constipation. Sadly, this is a side effect of the modern diet that is becoming more prevalent.

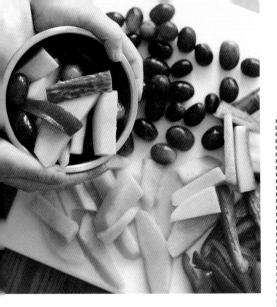

## fruit and vegetables

Everyone knows that it is recommended to eat at least 5 fruits and vegetables a day, but perhaps not everyone realizes that this includes frozen, dried, and canned fruit. The average fruit and vegetable consumption among children is less than 2 servings a day—a long way from the recommended 5.

Fruit and vegetables are a great source of vitamins, minerals, and fiber. Children need them in their diet to help boost their immune system. Fruits that are especially rich in immune-boosting vitamin C include oranges, kiwi fruit, strawberries, and raspberries. It is also believed that eating fresh fruits and vegetables during childhood can help reduce the risk of cancer, heart disease, and stroke later in life.

Every packed lunch should ideally have at least 1 piece of fruit and at least 1 serving of vegetables. To help your child reach the target of at least 5 servings a day, make sure that at each meal and snack he/she is eating 1 serving of fruit or vegetables. To make it more interesting, serve different colors each time and let your child be involved in the preparation.

### *fruit & vegetable requirement*

Children need 3 servings of vegetables a day. A rough guide to 1 serving of vegetables is approximately the amount a child can hold in his/her hand:

**Vegetables**
For children aged 5–8 years, a serving is:
- 1 small carrot
- ⅓ cup vegetables (such as sweetcorn, celery, broccoli)
- 3 or 4 cherry tomatoes

For children aged 9–11 years, a serving is:
- 1 carrot
- ½ cup vegetables (such as sweetcorn, celery, broccoli)
- 5–6 cherry tomatoes

Children need 2–3 servings of fruit a day. A rough guide to 1 serving of fruit is approximately the amount a child can hold in his/her hand:

**Fruit**
For children aged 5–8 years, a serving is:
- 1 small fruit, such as a plum
- 1 kiwi fruit
- 1 small orange or clementine
- 6 strawberries
- a big handful of dried fruit
  ½ cup canned fruit
- ½ cup fruit juice

For children aged 9–11 years, a serving is:
- 1–2 small fruits like a plum, kiwi fruit, or clementine
- 10 strawberries
- a big handful of dried fruit
  ¾ cup canned fruit
- ¾ cup fruit juice

*Note: Raw fruit and vegetables have the most nutrients.

## calcium

Calcium is vital for healthy bones and teeth and is also involved in maintaining normal nerve and muscle function. Good calcium-rich foods include cheese, milk, yogurt, soy milk (if fortified with calcium), soy yogurt, sardines (with bones mashed in), and nuts (especially almonds). These foods are also high in protein.

Try as much as possible to avoid buying yogurts that are high in sugar, and avoid any with artificial sweeteners, colors and flavors. Try adding fresh fruit purees to give flavor. Homemade milkshakes or smoothies can also be a great way of adding calcium to your child's diet, especially if he/she is not keen on drinking milk or eating yogurt. Avoid any cheese brands that are marketed at children. Although they contain the same amount of calcium as real cheese, they are also often laden with additives and salt.

### *calcium requirement*

Children need 3 servings of foods from the milk, yogurt, and cheese group or other high calcium foods a day. See below for guides:

For children aged 5–8 years, a serving is:
- ¾ cup of milk
- ¾ cup yogurt
- a handful of cheese
- 1–2 tinned sardines (with bones mashed)

For children aged 9–11 years, a serving is:
- 1 cup of milk
- 1 cup of yogurt
- a handful of cheese
- 2 tinned sardines (with bones mashed)

## salt

Children are vulnerable to the side effects of too much salt or sodium in their diet, and should limit their intake. Salt is made up of sodium and chloride, 1 g of sodium is equivalent to about 2.5 g of salt. Where do we get sodium? In addition to adding salt at the table with a salt shaker, the obvious foods that have high sodium levels include chips and salted nuts. Sodium is also found in foods where you might not expect it, such as cereal bars, baked goods, canned foods (tuna in brine, soup, canned vegetables), smoked and cured meats (salami, bacon), and sauces (soy sauce, tomato ketchup, pasta sauce). Make sure you check the labels on these foods.

### sodium intake

Aim to keep sodium intake below the following:
for children aged 4–6 years:
1900 mg sodium per day
for children aged 7–10 years:
2200 mg per day
for children aged 11–14 years:
2300 mg per day

**Note:** Sadly, the reality is that many children in the USA are actually eating far in excess of the recommended intake. Looking carefully at labels on food can help guide you in making lower sodium choices. Sodium is listed on the food label as milligrams (mg) sodium per serving. Look for lower sodium food choices labeled low sodium, sodium-free, or very low sodium, these have less than 140 mg per serving. Foods labeled reduced sodium contain at least 25% less sodium than the regular product but still may contain a considerable amount of sodium, so use these in moderation.

## sugar

Like salt, too much refined sugar can be bad for children. Refined sugar provides very little nutrition, except calories. Unrefined sugar (natural brown sugar) does provide a few nutrients, but should still be kept to a sensible limit. A much healthier option is food that naturally contains sugar, like fresh fruit, which also contains fiber and vitamins to promote health.

There are lots of obvious foods that contain sugar, but there are also many foods that contain hidden sugars. You will probably be surprised to learn that many yogurts (especially brands marketed at children), breakfast cereals, and some canned vegetables contain quite a lot of sugar.

It is believed that too much sugar in your child's diet can cause swings in blood sugar levels, which can lead to poor concentration, bad behavior, and low energy levels, although this is still being researched. It is also a major contributor to tooth decay and obesity. The World Health Organisation recommends that adults and children should get no more than 10 per cent of their calories from sugar.

Keep your child's sugar intake to a minimum by giving him/her lots of fresh fruit and vegetables. You can also make cakes and cookies at home, so you know how much sugar has gone into the food. Many recipes can easily have the amount of sugar reduced. If you want to give your child a piece of cake or a cereal bar that contains sugar, it is best to give this as part of a meal. This is because during a meal the amount of saliva in the mouth increases, therefore making it easier to wash the food, and sugar, away from the teeth.

Children don't need to have a sweet treat in their packed lunch every day—vary it with plain yogurt mixed with granola, pureed fruit, or a handful of dried fruits. Even though dried fruits contain high amounts of natural sugar, they are slow-releasing especially when combined with a slow-release carbohydrate (see page 121 for Apricot Slices as an example).

Try not to add sugar to food unless absolutely necessary. Even fruits that may taste slightly sour to you, can taste sweet to children, especially if they are not used to eating lots of sweet foods. Limit processed foods that may contain lots of unnecessary sugar and keep to low-sugar snacks, like rice cakes, plain crackers, fruit, vegetables, and popcorn.

### sugar intake

Sugar is added to many foods in different forms. Try to avoid processed foods with high-sugar content.

Check the ingredient list on food labels for the following—sucrose, glucose, dextrose, fruit syrup, fructose or high fructose corn syrup and glucose. These are all forms of sugar.

# fats

Children need some fat for optimum health. It is particularly important that a child's diet includes "good" fats, but limits the "bad" fats. The best fats are monounsaturated and polyunsaturated fats. Monounsaturated fats are found in olive oil, almonds, almond oil, peanuts, hazelnuts, avocados, and olives. These are believed to help keep cholesterol levels low and reduce the risk of heart disease and cancer in later life. Many of these foods are also good sources of vitamin E, an important antioxidant.

Polyunsaturated fats include omega-3 and omega-6 essential fatty acids. Omega-3 fatty acids provide the essential fatty acid alpha linolenic acid and are found in walnuts, walnut oil, flax (or linseed), and oily fish (mackerel, herring, sardines, salmon, fresh tuna, and trout). These fats are very important for brain development, and some studies have suggested that poor concentration in schoolchildren may be linked to low intakes of these omega-3 fatty acids in their diet. Omega-6 fatty acids are most common in nuts, seeds, and their oils (e.g. sunflower oil, sesame oil) and contain the essential fatty acid linoleic acid. They are also important in many aspects of growth and brain development. Omega-6 fats should be balanced with omega-3 fats and not eaten excessively.

Saturated and trans fats are the ones to minimize or avoid. Saturated fats are found naturally in animal product, such as meat and butter, whereas trans fats are formed when healthy unsaturated oils are changed during hydrogenation, a process that is used to harden liquid vegetable oils into solids. These fats are often found in margarines and many processed foods, such as cakes, cookies and chips. Trans fats are no longer being used in many processed foods or foods prepared in restaurants. They must now be declared on a food label. When shopping, look for foods that are free from trans fats. A small amount of saturated fat in the diet is reasonable. High intakes of these fats (saturated and trans) are associated with the development of atherosclerosis (fatty deposits in the arteries), which can lead to heart disease and stroke. They may also be a risk factor in the development of other diseases, such as cancer and, when combined with a high calorie diet, obesity.

To help increase the good fats in your child's diet, try to cook with olive or canola oil, and use other nut and seed oils, such as walnut or flaxseed oil, to make salad dressings. Flaxseed oil is available in some supermarkets and healthfood stores. Try adding it to smoothies or yogurts. Also, including oily fish in your child's diet each week provides a good source of protein as well as a healthy boost of omega-3 fats.

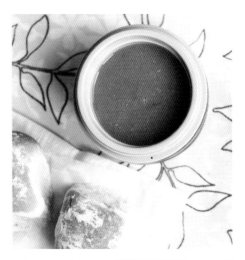

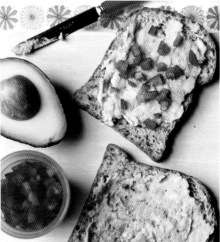

## *fat intake*

Try to avoid adding excess fat to your child's diet, aim to use small amounts of healthy fats for cooking and spreads and include at least 1 serving a week (60–80 g) of oily fish and some of the foods listed below.

For children aged 5–8 years try to include the following each day:
- 1 tablespoon nuts and seeds
- 2 teaspoons nut or seed oils

For children aged 9–11 years try to include the following each day:
- 1 heaped tablespoon nuts and seeds
- 1 tablespoon nut or seed oils

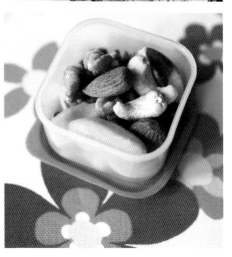

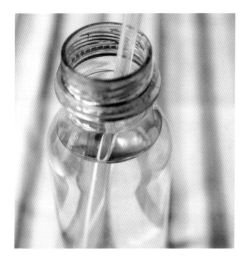

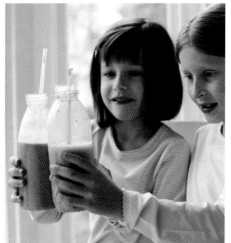

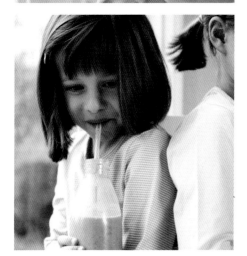

## what to drink

When it comes to drinks, water is best. Children should take a bottle of water to school with them every day. Most children do not drink enough water and a high percentage of schoolchildren are dehydrated. When your child becomes dehydrated, it has a negative impact on his/her ability to concentrate in class. Most schools have water fountains and some teachers are recognizing that it is a good idea to allow children to keep bottles of water in their classroom. Encourage your child to drink water at school.

If children are reluctant to drink plain water, which is often the case, or if they have become used to drinking juices or sodas, you will need to work hard at encouraging them to drink it. Only give them water to take to school, with the occasional fruit smoothie or juice in their lunchbox. Pack fun-coloured straws and, if that doesn't work, fill up bottles with water and then ask your child to decorate them with his/her favorite stickers.

If you want to give your child fresh fruit juice, pack a small bottle or juice box with his/her lunch, but explain that he/she will still need to drink water during the rest of the day. Water should be the drink children automatically ask for when they are thirsty. You should only give them fruit juice occasionally. Children can easily consume large amounts of juice, which will reduce their appetite for other foods and provide excess calories. A good guide is to limit to one drink of juice a day.

## why water?

**Children need water to:**
- help keep them hydrated
- help with concentration and memory
- help aid digestion and absorption
- help prevent constipation
- eliminate toxins from the body
- maintain body temperature (for example, if children have been playing sport on a hot day, they need water to help their bodies cool down).

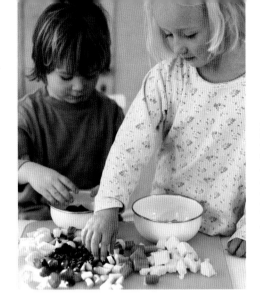

## how to involve your children

There is no doubt in my mind that children who help with choosing food and preparing it are more likely to enjoy eating it. Believe it or not, involving them can actually help you too, and doesn't always involve a lot of mess.

Children can help with simple tasks that will save you time and make them feel involved, such as peeling and washing carrots, counting out fruit and putting it into containers, and choosing dried fruits and mixing them together.

At weekends, when you have more time to spend in the kitchen, ask them to help make food that can go in the freezer. Tarts, muffins, fruit slices, cakes, and cookies can all be made and frozen, allowing you to take one out at a time to put in your child's packed lunch. You can even put frozen food into your child's packed lunch—it should have thawed by lunchtime, and it will help to keep other foods in the lunchbox fresh.

If your child is particularly fussy about food, come to an arrangement where there may be something in the lunchbox that he/she chooses and something that you choose. Write the occasional note and put it inside your child's lunchbox so he/she knows you are thinking of them. Write something funny that will make your child relax and perhaps encourage him/her to eat their lunch. Help your child enjoy lunchtime, so that it's something to look forward to rather than a chore. It may take a bit of effort on your part, but the end result is very satisfying for both parent and child.

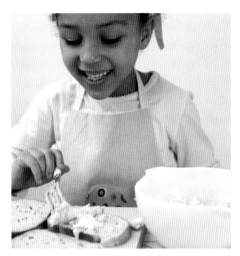

### growing alfalfa sprouts

Growing your own cress is just one inventive way to get your children involved with making their own packed lunches (see opposite).

### how to grow alfalfa sprouts

1 Purchase a packet of seeds from your local garden center or supermarket.

2 Find a suitable container and line it with a paper towel, cotton wool, or a thick layer of seed compost.

3 Moisten the paper towel with water and sprinkle the seeds over the top.

4 Cover with a paper towel until the seeds start to germinate, then remove.

5 It's important to keep the sprouts moist, so sprinkle with water when needed.

6 Cut the sprouts with scissors when it's about 2 inches high. The sprouts should take up to 14 days to reach this height.

7 Put the sprouts in a sandwich of your choice (see egg and sprout sandwich idea on page 32).

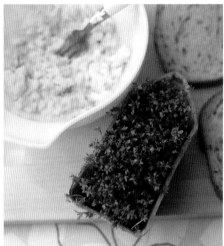

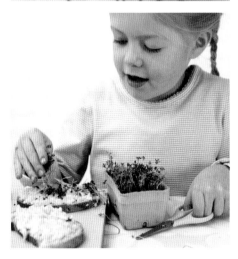

# the perfect lunchbox

You are certainly not alone if you struggle to think of things to put into your child's lunchbox. Once you have managed to gather together some bits and pieces, you may still be left wondering whether the lunch will provide your child with enough of the right nutrients. You may also be unsure as to whether he/she will actually eat the food that you have given him/her.

Sadly, studies have shown that many lunchboxes contain double the recommended daily amount of sugar and nearly half the safe daily intake for salt and saturated fats. Popular items found in children's lunchboxes include chocolate bars and packets of chips, and very few contain fresh fruit.

A good lunchbox should provide your child with enough energy to sustain him/her all afternoon. It should provide approximately one third of the recommended daily energy needs, as well as approximately one third of the daily protein, carbohydrate, fiber, vitamin, and mineral requirements. Making a balanced lunchbox is surprisingly easy to achieve. Opposite is a simple checklist to get you started.

- **fruit**
1 serving of fresh or dried fruit

- **vegetables**
1 serving of vegetables or salad (e.g. carrots, celery, bell peppers, cucumber)

- **dairy**
1 item from this group, such as cheese, yogurt, milk OR alternatively another calcium-rich food, such as calcium-fortified soya, tofu, canned fish, like pilchards and sardines (the edible bones are a good source of calcium), and nuts.

- **protein**
1 serving of food from the meat, poultry, fish, dry beans, eggs, and nuts group of protein-rich foods.

- **carbohydrate**
1 or more servings of foods from the bread, cereals, pasta, and rice group.

- **drink**
A drink—approximately 6–8 oz. This should preferably be water.

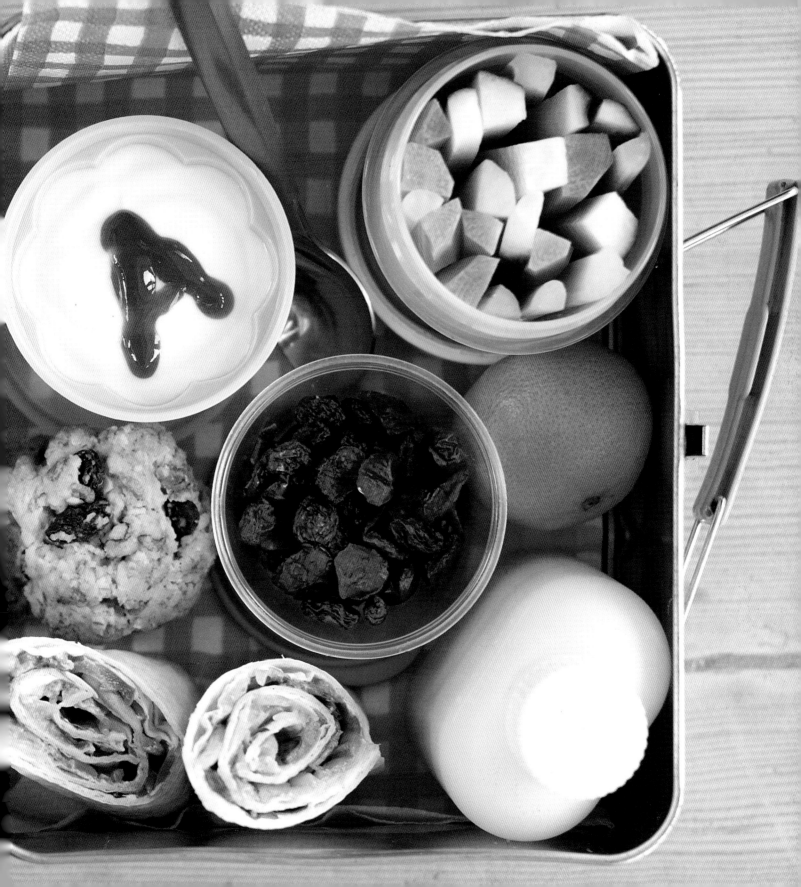

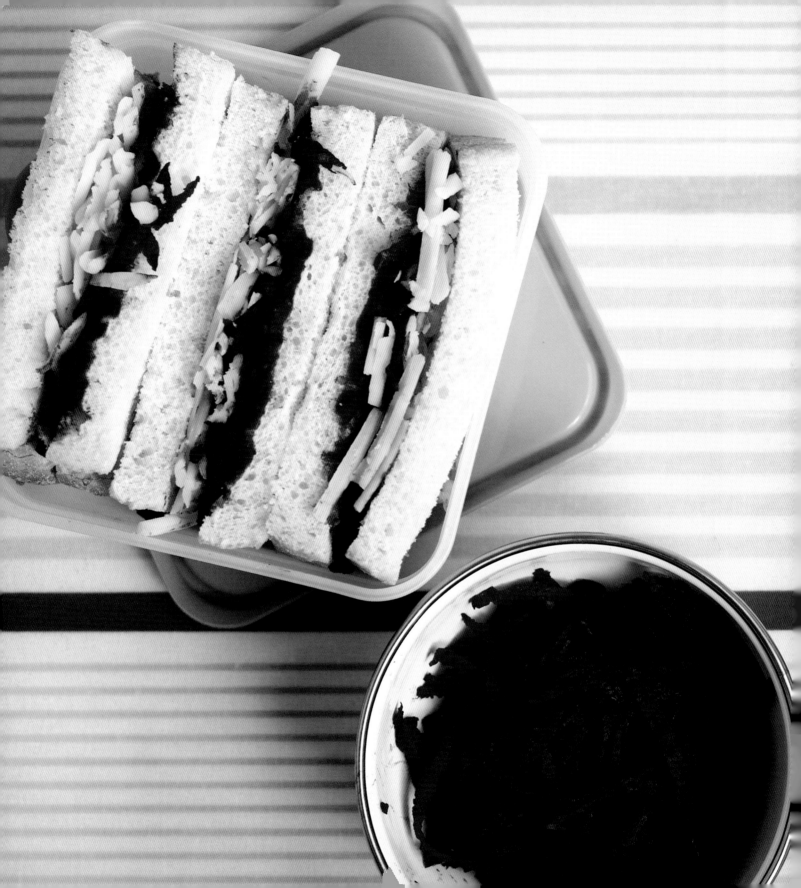

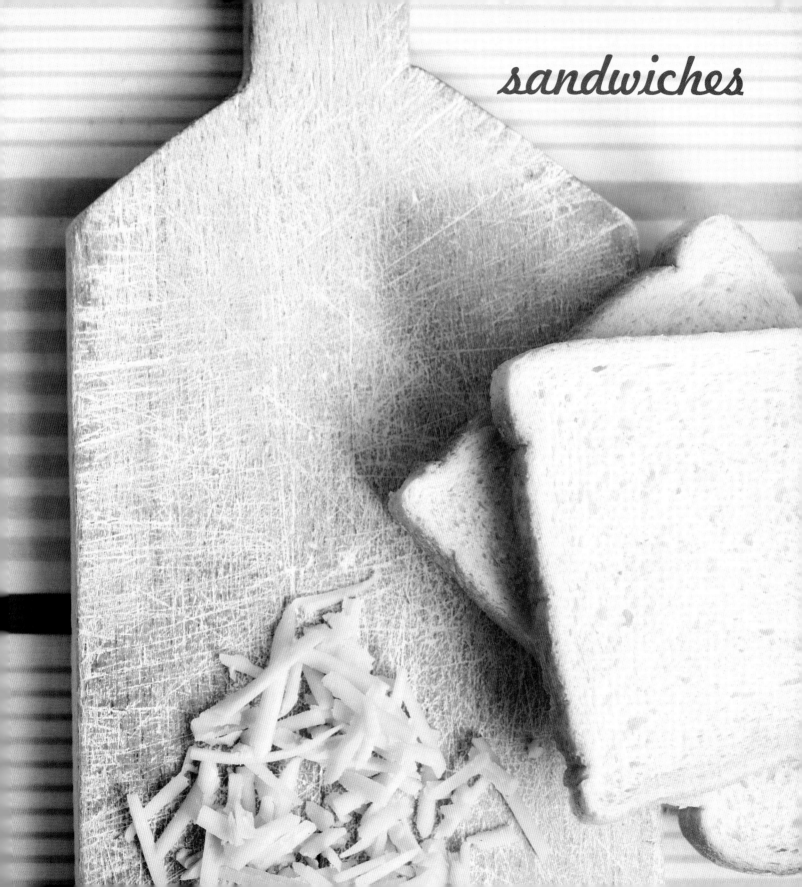

sandwiches

# breads

There are hundreds of different types of bread available in supermarkets today. It is no longer just a case of choosing between a white, wholewheat, or brown loaf. There are breads made from mixed grains, those that have been bran-enriched or fortified with vitamins and minerals, as well as fruit breads, seed breads, and nut breads. Bread also comes sliced, unsliced, wrapped, unwrapped, part-baked, and frozen.

There are different shaped breads, including the braided challah, fat Italian breads, torpedo-shaped ryes and pumpernickel, all sorts of rolls and buns, and, of course, your basic sandwich-type loaf. There are also baguettes and croissants, pita bread, ciabatta and focaccia, bagels, pretzels, and nan. The choice is enormous, and they are all good for children.

If your child demands white bread sandwiches, my advice is to persevere and slowly introduce your child to different breads. It is our job, as parents, to encourage our children to try different food.

White bread is made with white flour, which has had most of its fiber and some of its minerals and vitamins removed, and has sometimes been bleached or refined. It is fine to include some white bread in your child's diet, especially since it's often been fortified with calcium and niacin (a vitamin that aids the removal of toxic chemicals from the body), but make sure you also introduce other breads to your child's lunchbox. As a general guide, children over the age of 5 can have two thirds wholewheat or brown bread and one third white bread in their diet.

The sandwich recipes in the following chapter do not list the type of bread that should be used—on the whole, it is up to you to choose. Occasionally, suggestions have been made where a particular bread may work best.

## ▪ loaves—wholewheat, seeded, herb & tomato bread
Experiment with different types of bread each week; your child will enjoy his/her sandwiches more as a result. You may discover that your child will eat items in bread, such as tomatoes, that he/she wouldn't usually eat raw.

## ▪ pita bread
This is a flat bread traditionally from Greece and the Middle East. Children love pita breads for their pocket-like effect, and they often come in small sizes as well as large. Children particularly like them lightly toasted before they are filled.

## ▪ tortilla wraps
Made from wheat flour, these are ideal for wrapping soft ingredients, like cream cheese and peanut butter, and are easy for children to eat.

## ▪ rolls
Available in many varieties (white, brown, topped with seeds) and different shapes and sizes, you will often find that children are happier with small soft rolls because they are easier for them to eat.

## ▪ French bread & Italian bread
Some children find French bread takes too long to eat because of its hard outer crust, and don't finish it. It requires quite a lot of chewing, so children often get bored and leave their half-eaten sandwiches. But Italian bread has a softer crust, which children will more easily accept, so for lunchboxes, Italian bread is probably the one to choose.

## ▪ bagels
There are a variety of different bagel flavors available, and they are popular with children because of their chewy texture.

## ▪ ciabatta
A crusty white bread often identified by its shape, which resembles a flattened slipper, and thus the meaning of the word "ciabatta" in Italian. The great thing about ciabatta is that you can often buy it part-baked, which is ideal for keeping in the freezer until you need it.

## ▪ focaccia
A soft white Italian bread made with white flour and olive oil, often topped with onions, herbs, or other foodstuffs. It looks a bit like a thick pizza base.

## ▪ fruit bread & raisin bread
These are quite popular among young children because they have a hint of sweetness. Try spreading these breads with cream cheese.

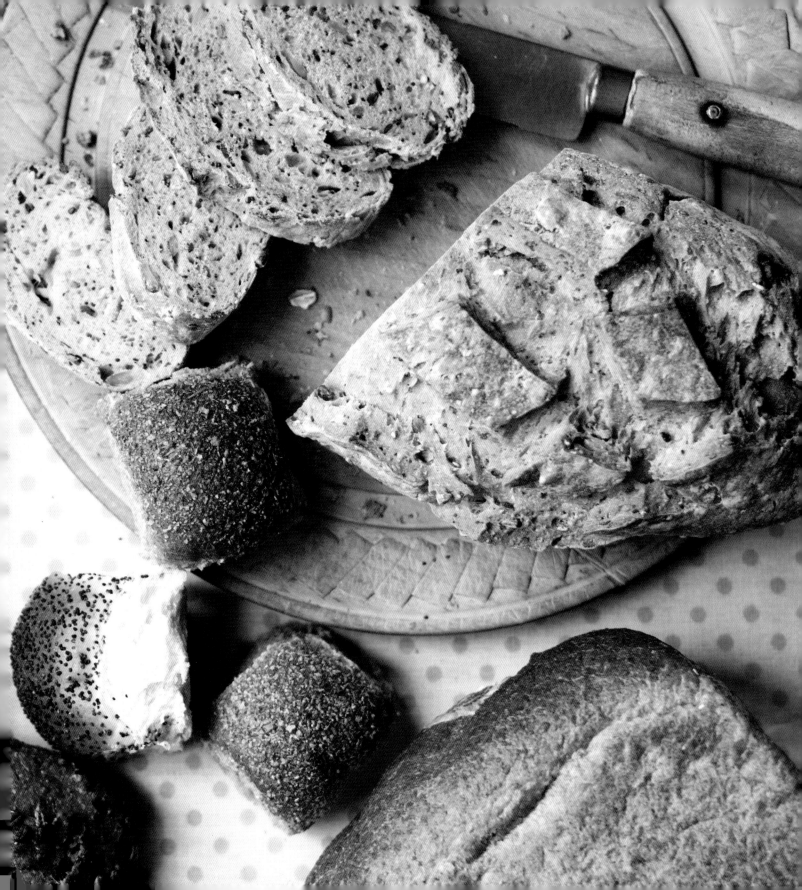

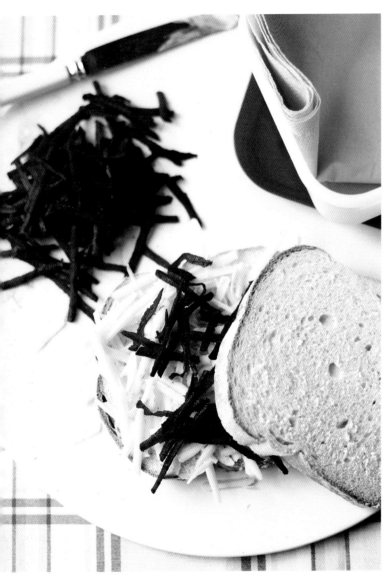

# cheese sandwiches

### cheddar with scallions & tomato

Grate a chunk of cheddar into a bowl, add ¼ scallion (finely chopped) and 1 ripe tomato (finely chopped). Mix the ingredients together and put into 2 rolls or pitas of your choice.

### ploughman's

Most children love this popular combination, and it's healthy for them. Put a big handful of grated cheddar into a roll or your choice, add 1 teaspoon chutney, 1 chopped tomato, and top with a handful of finely chopped lettuce.

### cheese & beet

Thinly slice a small piece of cheddar and place onto your chosen bread. Top with an equal amount of thinly sliced raw beet. You can also grate both of these if you think your child would prefer it.

### cheese & apple

Grate a chunk of your child's favorite hard cheese and mix it with grated apple, 1 chopped scallion, a squeeze of lemon, and a little mayonnaise. This combination is particularly good in wholewheat bread or rolls. If you want to add a bit more protein, you could also add a few chopped nuts.

### Greek sandwiches

Mix together some crumbled feta cheese with 3–4 black olives (pits removed) and a chopped ripe tomato. Spread onto your chosen bread.

### cream cheese & spinach

Spread some cream cheese onto a flour tortilla, top with 1 handful of washed baby spinach leaves (pick off any tough stalks), and then carefully roll the tortilla. Cut into 3 pieces, so that you have 3 easy-to-hold sandwiches.

**note:** all sandwiches make 1 unless otherwise stated.

### cream cheese & sun-dried tomatoes

Spread some cream cheese onto your chosen bread, and top with 1–2 finely chopped sun-dried tomatoes.

### cream cheese & red bell pepper

Spread some cream cheese onto your chosen bread and then scatter ¼ red bell pepper (finely chopped) over it. Alternatively, use a roasted red bell pepper from a jar, slice, and scatter it over the cheese.

### cream cheese & pesto

Spread some cream cheese onto your chosen bread and then spread a small amount of red or green pesto on top.

### cream cheese & pear

Spread some cream cheese onto your chosen bread and then thinly slice ½ pear and cover with a little lemon juice. Put the pear on top of the cheese.

### cream cheese & cucumber

Spread some cream cheese onto your chosen bread and top with thinly sliced cucumber.

### cream cheese & avocado

Spread some cream cheese onto your chosen bread, top with ½ avocado (sliced or roughly mashed with a few drops of lemon juice to stop it turning brown), and sprinkle with a few poppy seeds, if you like. Grated carrot and cream cheese also make a good combination.

### cottage cheese & pineapple

Mix together 2 tablespoons cottage cheese with a few pieces of chopped canned pineapple. Spoon onto your chosen bread.

### cottage cheese & fruit

Mix together 2 tablespoons cottage cheese with a few raisins and finely chopped dried apricots—or any other dried fruits. Spoon into a roll.

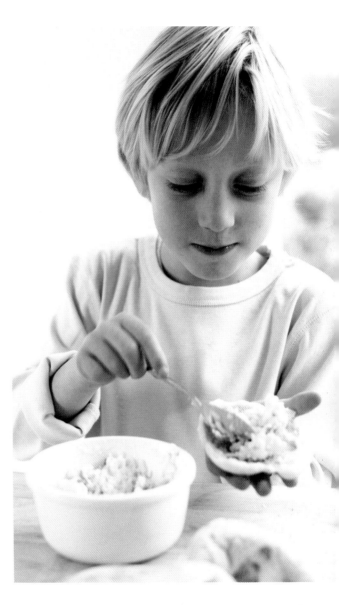

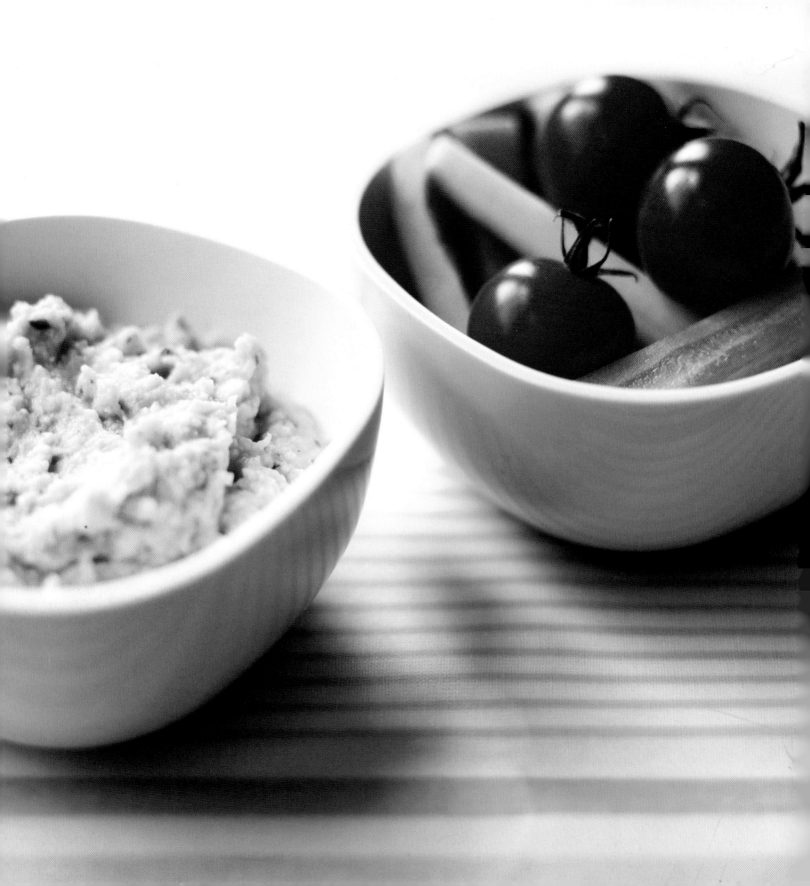

# hummus sandwiches

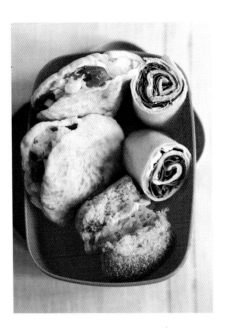

You can either make your own hummus or buy it. Avoid buying low-fat hummus because it often contains hydrogenated fats, which can raise cholesterol levels in the blood and are best avoided. You can combine hummus with all kinds of ingredients to add flavor and texture and then spread onto sandwiches, or serve as a dip with vegetable sticks.

## hummus & grated carrot

Spread some hummus onto your chosen bread, and top with a peeled and grated carrot.

## hummus & grated cheddar

Spread some hummus onto your chosen bread, and add a handful of grated cheddar cheese.

## hummus & avocado

Spread some hummus onto your chosen bread. Mash ½ ripe avocado with a few drops of lemon juice to prevent discoloration. Spread the avocado on top of the hummus.

## hummus & beet

Spread some hummus onto your chosen bread, and grate a little raw beet over the top.

## hummus, tomatoes, & lettuce

Spread some hummus onto your chosen bread, and top with slices of tomato and lettuce leaves.

If you want to make your own homemade hummus, see page 92.

**nutrition tip** Even if your child is not vegetarian, try to include some vegetable protein foods in his/her diet, like chickpeas, since they provide a great type of fiber that is beneficial to the digestive system.

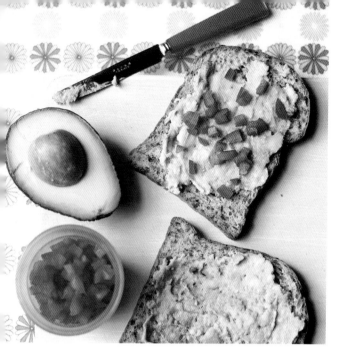

# vegetarian sandwiches

If you are feeding your child a vegetarian diet, you need to make sure he/she gets all the essential nutrients usually provided in meat.

## avocado & red bell pepper

Mash ½ ripe avocado with a little lemon juice, and spread onto your chosen bread. Finely chop ¼ bell pepper (orange, yellow, and red are sweeter than green) and sprinkle it over the top of the avocado. Alternatively, use a chopped roasted red bell pepper from a jar, sliced.

## falafel in pita

Falafel is best served in pita, and is easy to eat and tastes great. This is a very quick and simple version of falafel, and is a good way to encourage your children to eat chickpeas.

**makes** 12

2 tablespoons olive oil

1 small onion, chopped

1 garlic clove, peeled and crushed

2 x 15-oz. cans chickpeas, washed and drained

1 teaspoon ground cumin

1 teaspoon ground coriander

a handful of freshly chopped cilantro or mint

2 tablespoons mango chutney

freshly ground black pepper

flour, lightly seasoned with salt and pepper

lettuce, shredded (optional)

1 tomato, sliced (optional)

Heat 1 tablespoon of the olive oil in a skillet, add the onion and garlic, and fry very gently until soft for approximately 5 minutes. Tip the onion and garlic into the bowl of a food processor, add the chickpeas, cumin, and ground coriander, then roughly whiz together.

Add the fresh cilantro and mango chutney, and season with ground black pepper.

Mold the mixture into 12 balls and flatten into patty shapes. Dip them in the seasoned flour so they are lightly coated. Heat the remaining olive oil in the skillet and fry the falafels on medium heat for 3 minutes on each side until golden brown. Let cool, then put into pita breads with the lettuce, tomato, and extra mango chutney, if you like.

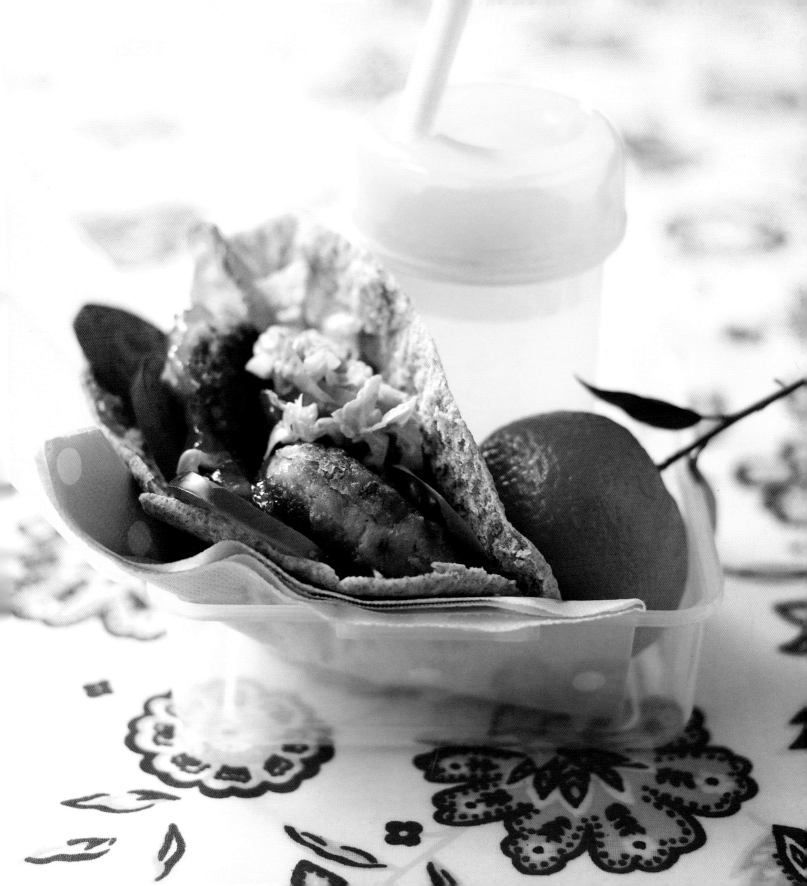

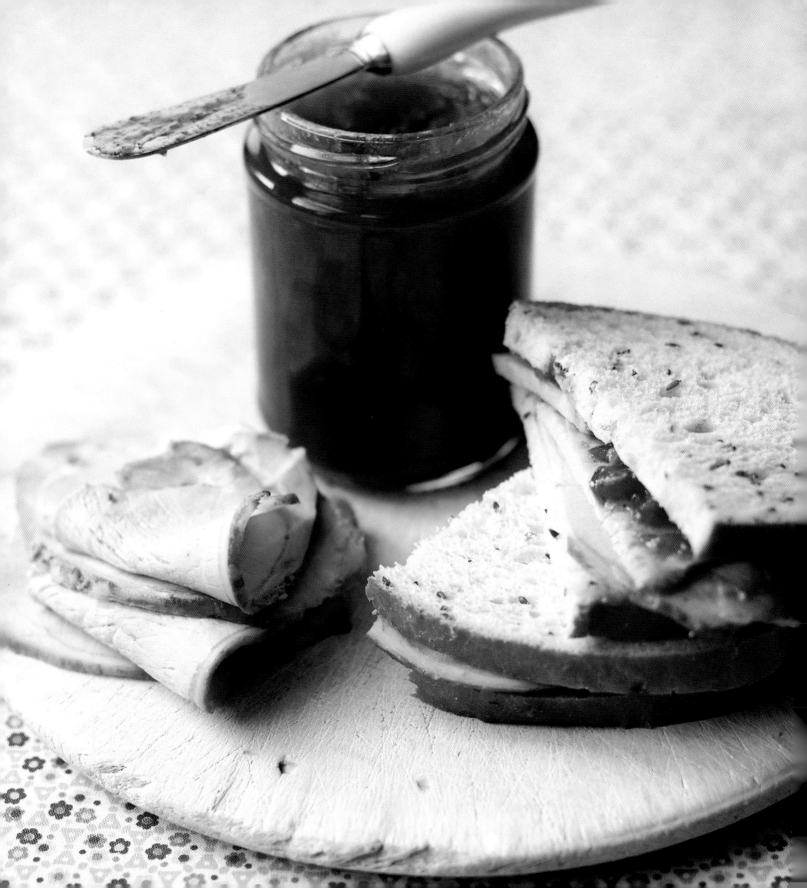

# roast meats & bacon

One great thing about having a roast at the weekend is that you should have some leftover cold meat, ideal for packed lunches at the beginning of the week. A slice of meat counts as 1 portion of your child's daily protein requirement (see page 7).

### roast beef with horseradish & cucumber

Some children love the taste of horseradish, others hate it and find it too hot. Spread a tiny amount of horseradish over your chosen bread, top with 2 pieces of roast beef and a few thin slices of cucumber.

### roast pork with apple sauce

Most children love this combination. Finely chop 2 slices of cooked pork and mix with 2 tablespoons apple sauce. Spoon the mixture into a roll. Alternatively, split the roll, spread with apple sauce and fill with the pork. The apple sauce adds a wonderful sweetness and helps to bind the pork together.

### roast pork with chutney

If your child likes chutney, mixing it with a cold meat is an easy Monday-morning sandwich filler. Spread some chutney onto your chosen bread and top with 2 slices of pork.

### lamb with mint jelly & baby spinach

This may not sound like one of your typical sandwich fillings, but it just makes sense to use up leftover meats and mix them with their natural accompaniments. Spread some mint jelly onto your chosen bread. Top with 2 slices of leftover lamb and some baby spinach leaves, which are a great source of iron.

### bacon with watercress & grated carrot

Finely chop 2 strips of fried bacon and put onto your chosen bread. Top with a handful of watercress and grated carrot.

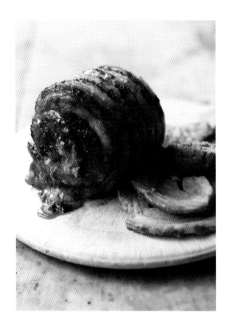

### blt

With this combination, it works best if all the ingredients are finely chopped and mixed together, especially for younger children. Older children can manage eating bigger pieces of bacon with sliced tomatoes and shredded lettuce. Put 2 strips fried bacon onto your chosen bread and top with slices of tomato and a little shredded lettuce.

### bacon with egg & tomato

Mash 1 hard-cooked egg (see page 32), spread onto 2 slices of bread, sprinkle with 2 finely chopped strips of fried bacon, and top with 1 ripe sliced tomato. This makes 2 sandwiches.

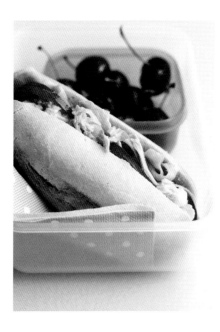

# ham & sausages

### ham with grated cheese

This is my middle daughter's all-round favorite sandwich, and she says it works best in a soft roll. Put 2 slices of ham into a roll and top with a handful of grated cheddar.

### ham with beet relish

Spread a little beet (or other) relish onto your chosen bread. Top with 2 slices of ham.

### ham with tomato & shredded lettuce

Put 2 slices of ham into a roll and add 1 thinly sliced tomato and a little shredded lettuce. This is easier for a child to eat in a roll, because the filling is less likely to fall out.

### cooked sausage & tomato

Thinly slice a cooked cold sausage lengthwise. Spread some tomato ketchup onto your chosen bread and top with the sausage slices and 1 sliced tomato.

### sausage & chutney

Thinly slice a cooked cold sausage. Spread some chutney onto your chosen bread and top with the sausage slices. Try the sesame seed sausages opposite if your child has a hankering for something a little more exciting than plain sausages (see page 73).

**nutrition tip** Always choose good -quality sausages; cheap sausages are packed with cheap fillers. For some extra-special sausages, try the sesame seed sausages on page 73. These are popular with adults, as well as children, and are perfect for birthday parties.

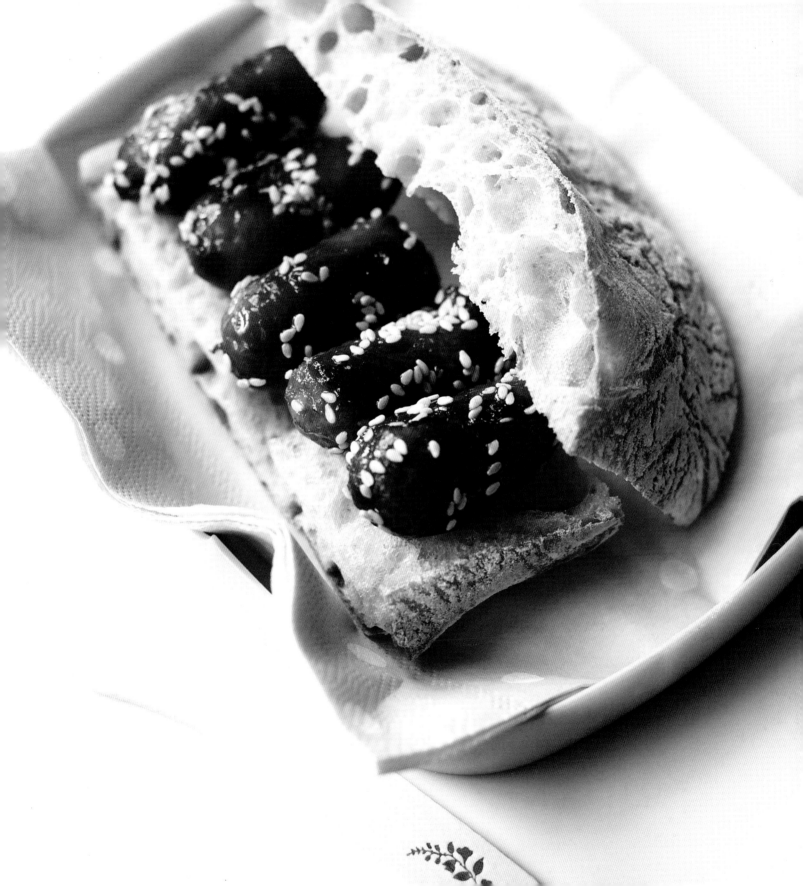

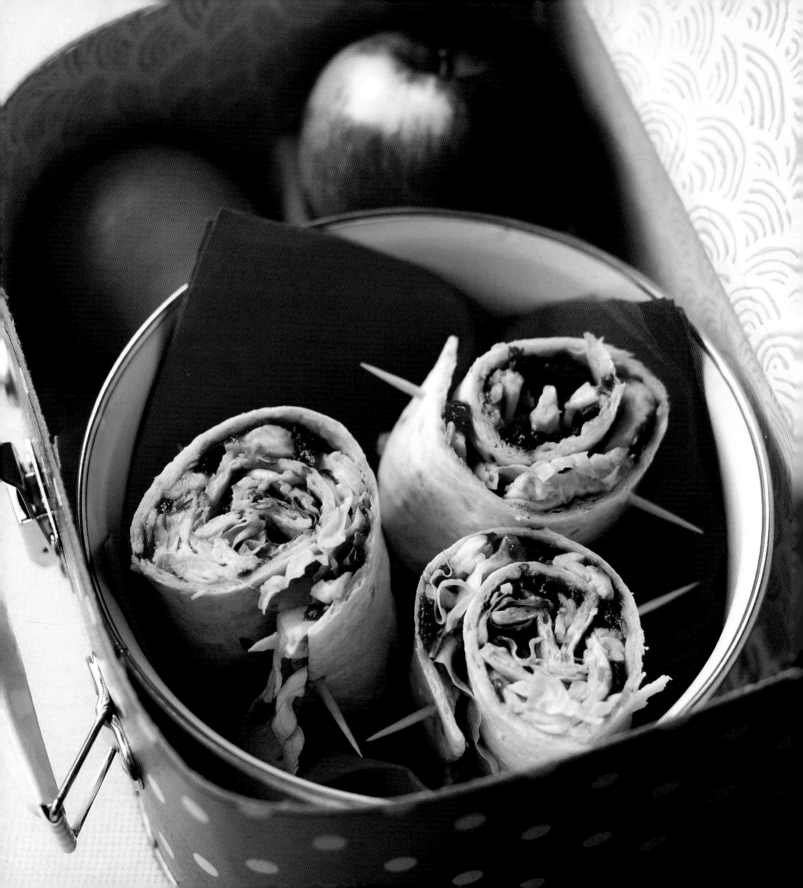

# chicken & turkey

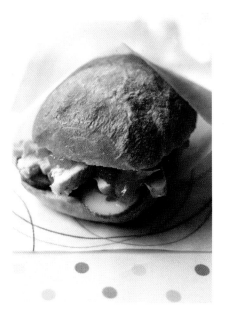

### chicken with mayonnaise, yogurt, raisins, & nuts

Finely chop 2 slices of cooked chicken breast and put into a bowl. Add a little mayonnaise, yogurt, a handful of raisins (or cranberries), and a handful of chopped nuts. Mix together and spoon into a pita bread.

### chicken with mango chutney & cucumber

Shred a little cooked chicken and put into a pita pocket or a roll, top with a spoonful of mango chutney, and some thinly sliced cucumber.

### turkey with scallions & apple sauce

Shred some cooked turkey meat. Spread a little apple sauce onto your chosen bread and scatter the turkey over it. Top with ¼ of a chopped scallion and cut into 2 sandwiches.

### turkey with cranberry sauce & lettuce

Shred some cooked turkey meat. Spread some cranberry sauce onto a wrap and top with the turkey and shredded lettuce. If you make these wraps the night before, place a toothpick through them to hold them together. Remove the toothpicks before packing your child's lunch, and roll the wraps up in greaseproof paper.

**nutrition tip** Turkey is a good source of zinc—a mineral that helps aid digestion and maintain a healthy immune system. It is also important for healthy skin.

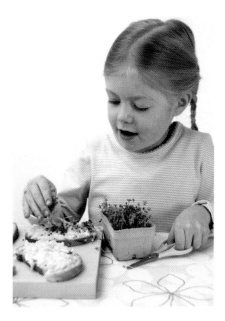

# egg sandwiches

### egg salad, with watercress or lettuce

Lightly mash a hard-cooked egg in a bowl. Add 2 teaspoons mayonnaise or salad dressing, and season with freshly ground black pepper. Mix together the ingredients, spoon onto your chosen bread, and add a handful of fresh watercress.

### egg & sprouts

Has your child ever grown alfalfa sprouts? It's fun and a great way to illustrate where food comes from. You will also find that your child is more willing to eat things that he/she has helped to grow (see page 13 for instructions).

Lightly mash a hard-cooked egg in a bowl. Add 2 teaspoons mayonnaise or salad dressing. Spoon the mixture onto your chosen bread. Add a handful of your homegrown fresh sprouts, cutting from the bottom.

### egg, bacon, & tomato sandwich for two

You do not need to add any mayonnaise or salad dressing, since the tomatoes add flavor and moisture. Fry 2 bacon strips until crisp. Cut into small pieces. Lightly mash 2 hard-cooked eggs in a bowl. Finely chop 2 ripe tomatoes and add to the egg along with the bacon. Mix together and then spoon onto your chosen bread.

### egg with red bell pepper & cucumber

Lightly mash a hard-cooked egg in a bowl. Add ¼ red bell pepper (finely chopped) to the bowl and a little finely chopped cucumber. Mix well, then spoon onto your chosen bread. You can thinly slice the pepper and cucumber if you prefer.

## how to hard cook eggs

Fill a saucepan three-quarters full with water and bring to a boil. Carefully add the eggs. Set the timer for 7 minutes (large eggs will need 8 minutes). Lift the eggs out of the saucepan with a slotted spoon. Run cold water over the eggs to stop them cooking and to help cool them down. Peel away the shell.

Most children like to eat hard-cooked eggs plain and often like to peel away the shell themselves. They make a great little lunchbox filler. If your child likes to eat his/her egg with some dressing, include a little blob of salad dressing or mayonnaise in a tub. Most brands of mayonnaise are made with pasteurized egg yolk, but always check the label. Add some bread and vegetable sticks to eat alongside an egg, and your child's packed lunch is ready.

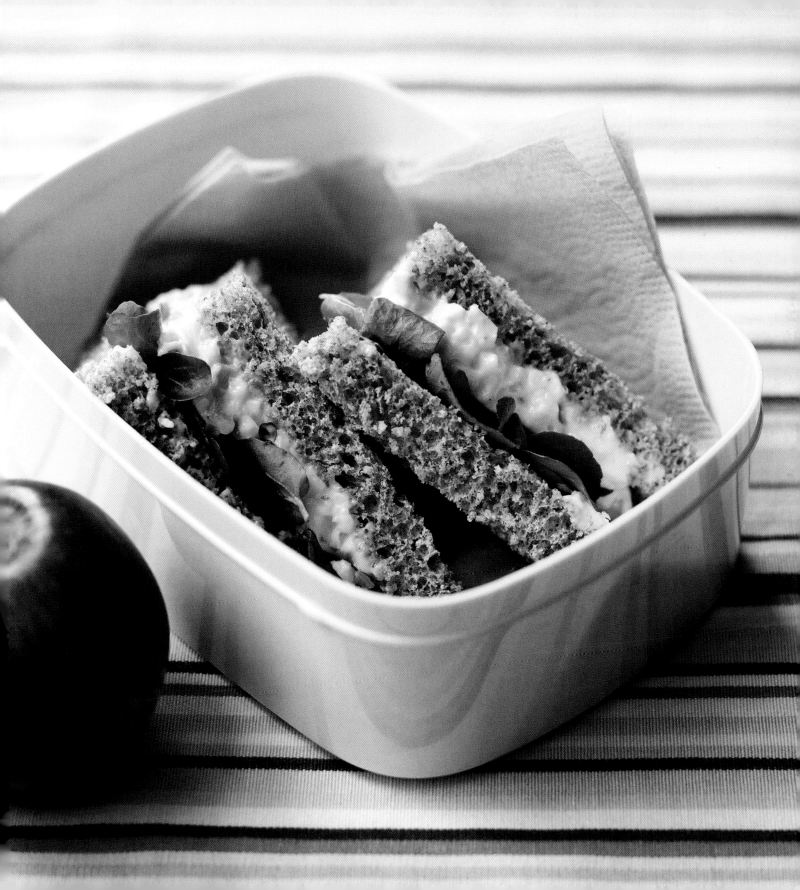

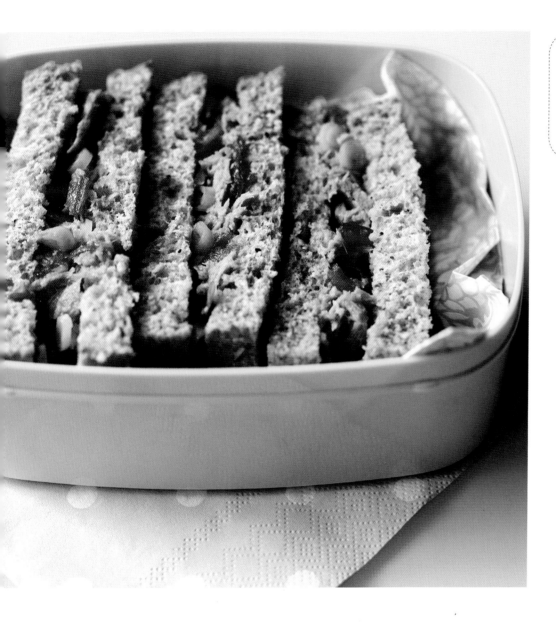

**nutrition tip** Poor diet has been linked to problems such as learning difficulties, hyperactivity, attention deficit hyperactive disorder (ADHD), depression, stress, and anxiety. It is therefore important that you offer your child a varied and healthy diet.

# fish sandwiches

Fish is something that children love or hate, but it's a good idea to make sure they have some in their diet. Tuna is the easiest option, but some children also love sardines and salmon, both of which are good cupboard standbys.

**note:** Drain all canned products before using.

## tuna salad with corn

This classic combination is liked by most children, and is very easy to make. Add a little mayonnaise to some canned tuna with a handful of canned or fresh cooked corn, and mix everything together. Spread onto your chosen bread.

## tuna with scallions & tomato

Mix together half a can of tuna with ¼ of a finely chopped scallion and 1 finely chopped ripe tomato. Spread onto your chosen bread.

## tuna with cream cheese & lettuce

Spread your chosen bread with cream cheese, top with a little canned tuna and shredded lettuce.

## tuna with cucumber

Mash some canned tuna, spread onto your chosen bread, and top with thinly sliced cucumber. Alternatively, mix the tuna with a little finely chopped cucumber. Canned salmon works well too.

## salmon with tomato ketchup & sprouts

Mash some boned canned red salmon with a little tomato ketchup. Spread onto wholewheat bread and sprinkle with lots of alfalfa sprouts (see page 13 on how to grow your own sprouts).

## sardines, lemon, & lettuce

Mash 2 canned sardines with a little lemon juice and spread onto your chosen bread. Top with a handful of shredded lettuce.

## shrimp salad & watercress

Shrimp are a good occasional treat. If you are using frozen ones, leave them to thaw first. Take a handful of cold cooked shrimp and mix them with a little mayonnaise and plain yogurt. Spread onto your chosen bread and top with watercress. This mixture is an acquired taste, but makes a great little sandwich filler.

## creamy smoked mackerel

Skin and flake smoked mackerel fillets, then mix with a little mayonnaise and Greek yogurt. Spread onto thick wholewheat bread and top with crisp lettuce leaves.

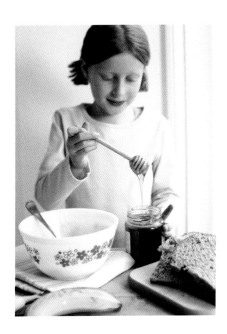

# easy sandwiches

If you're in a hurry, these quick sandwiches are ideal for occasional treats. They are firm favorites with children, and easy to eat if they're eager to go and play with their friends at lunchtime.

## peanut butter & banana

Spread some peanut butter onto your chosen bread and top with a thinly sliced banana.

## peanut butter with cucumber

Spread some peanut butter onto your chosen bread and top with thinly sliced cucumber.

## peanut butter with grated carrot & raisins

Thinly spread some peanut butter onto your chosen bread and top with grated carrot and a handful of raisins.

## jam & sliced banana

Spread some jam onto your chosen bread and top with sliced banana.

## mashed banana & honey

Mash a banana with a little lemon juice to stop the banana from going brown, add a little honey, and spread onto your chosen bread. Alternatively, spread a little honey in a roll and add the mashed banana.

## cheese & cucumber

Sprinkle some grated cheese onto your chosen bread and top with thinly sliced cucumber.

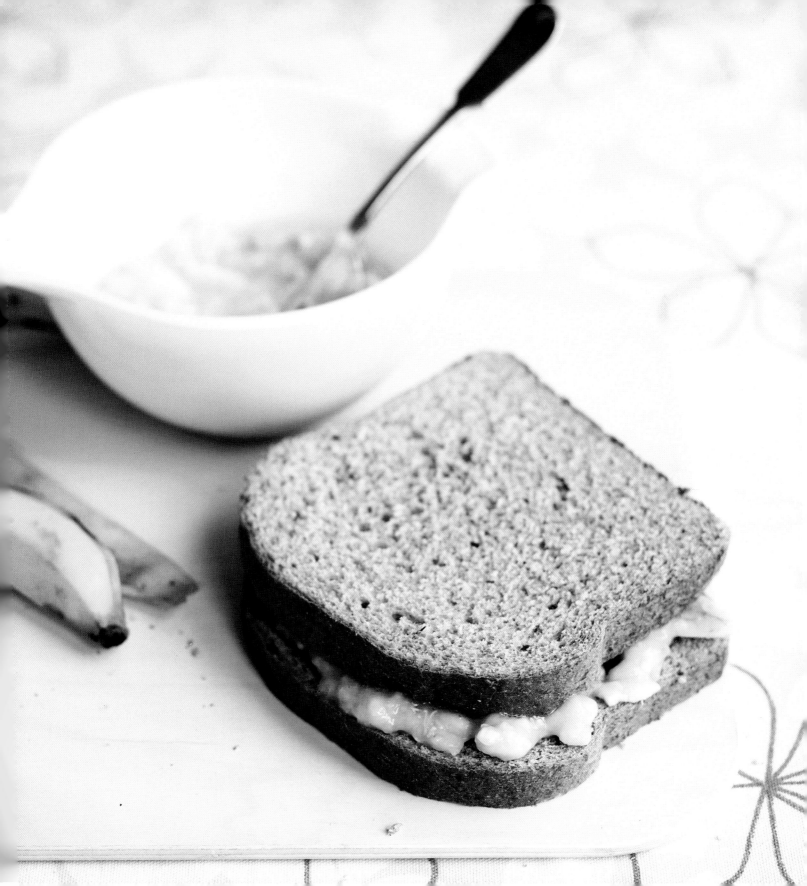

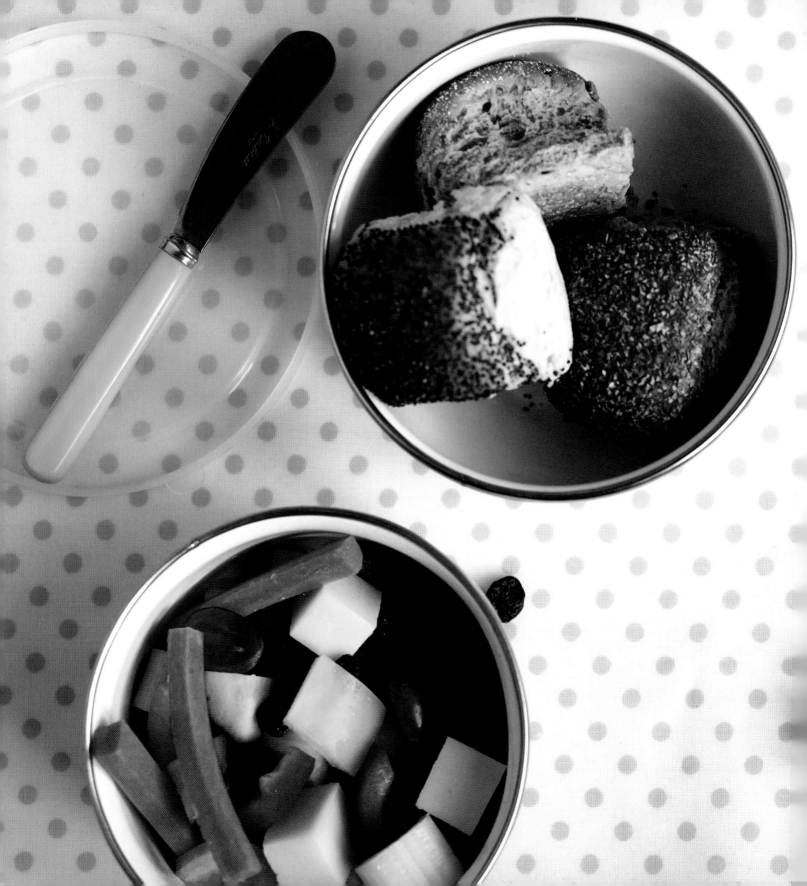

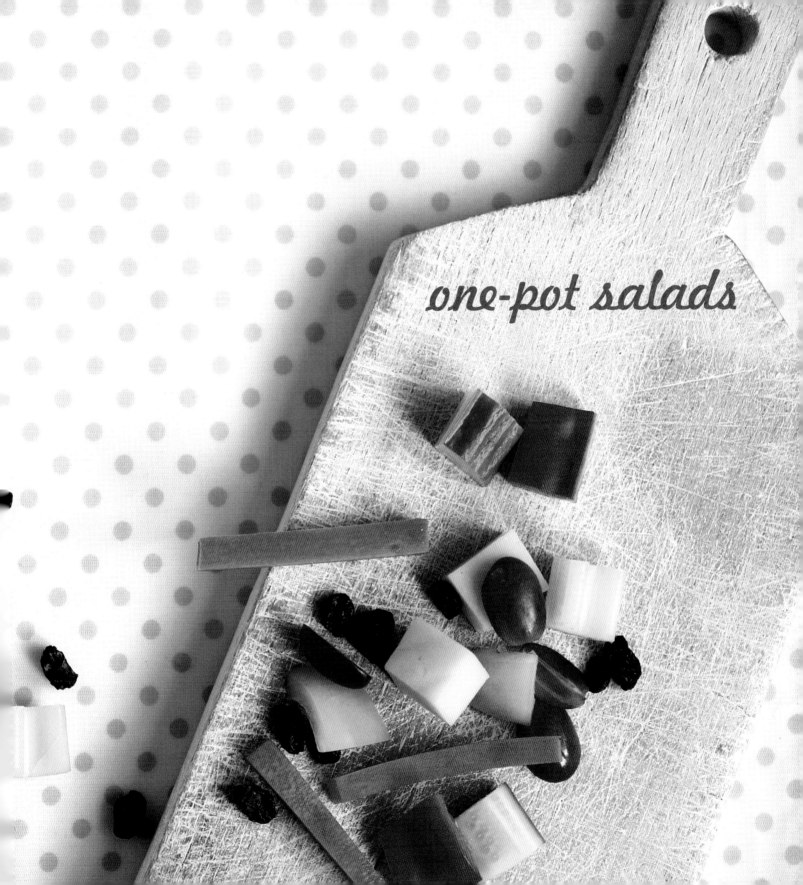

one-pot salads

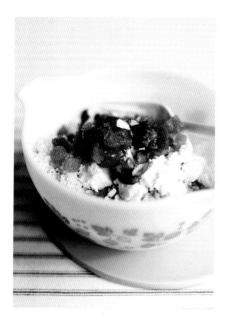

Try to vary between salads and sandwiches, so your child doesn't get bored with his/her lunch. You can add so many different things to couscous. It is a bit like pasta and changes flavor depending on the ingredients that you add to it. Don't forget to pop a spoon into the lunchbox with these salads.

# couscous

**nutrition tip** Semolina (made from the hard, outer part of wheat) is used to make couscous. It provides children with a great source of slow-release energy.

## couscous with feta

**serves** 2

½ cup couscous

½ cup boiling broth or water

a handful of dried apricots (about 4–5), finely chopped

a handful of almonds, finely chopped

a small chunk of feta cheese (about 2 oz.), crumbled

a small handful of fresh mint, finely chopped, or 1 teaspoon mint sauce

## couscous with tuna

**serves** 2

½ cup couscous

½ cup boiling broth or water

½ can tuna in sunflower oil, drained

a handful of black olives, finely chopped

4 cherry tomatoes, finely chopped

## couscous with cucumber

**serves** 2

½ cup couscous

½ cup boiling broth or water

¼ cucumber, finely chopped

a handful of fresh mint, finely chopped

2 ripe tomatoes, finely chopped

**dressing** (for all 3 recipes):

freshly squeezed juice of ½ lemon

3 tablespoons olive oil

1 teaspoon honey

Put the couscous into a bowl, pour a boiling broth over it, cover, and leave for 10 minutes.

Once the grains of couscous have absorbed all the liquid, fluff them up with a fork. Add the remaining ingredients from the recipe you've chosen, and mix together. Mix together the dressing ingredients and stir into the couscous. Keep chilled until ready to serve.

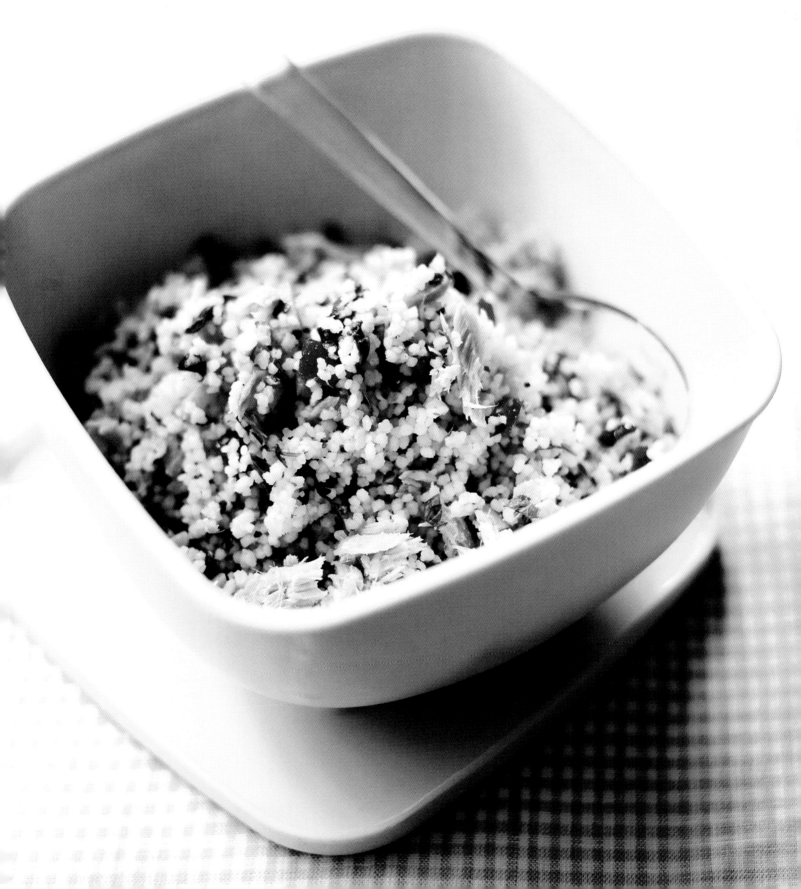

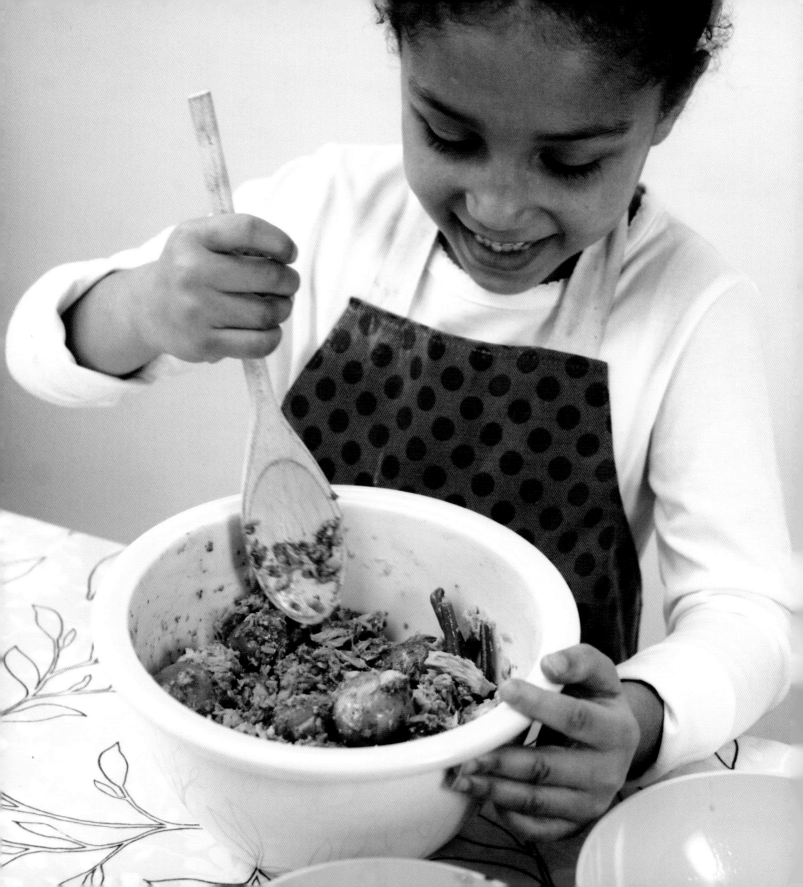

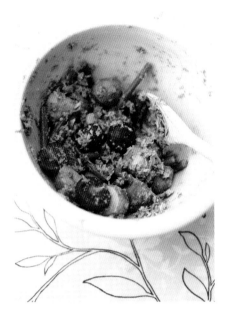

I always make these recipes for the whole family, hence why they both serve 4, but you can always cook half the amount or store half in the fridge for later. The Creamy Potato Salad is also good made with white cannellini beans instead of potatoes.

# potato salads

### creamy potato salad

**serves 4**

1 lb new potatoes, cut in half (about 3–4 cups)

2 tablespoons mayonnaise

1 tablespoon plain yogurt

a small handful of fresh mint or parsley, chopped

1–2 scallions, finely chopped

2 handfuls of cubed cheese, chopped ham, or cooked bacon (for protein)

freshly ground black pepper

Bring a small pan of water to a boil, add the potatoes and boil for 10–12 minutes until just cooked. Drain.

Mix together the mayonnaise, yogurt, and herbs in a bowl. Season with a little black pepper. Add the potatoes, scallions, and cheese.

Mix everything together, let cool, and store in the fridge until needed.

### potato, pesto, & tuna salad

**serves 4**

1 lb new potatoes, cut in half (about 3–4 cups)

2 large handfuls of green beans (about 5–6 oz.)

2 tablespoons green pesto

1 tablespoon olive oil

1 cup canned tuna, drained

a handful of cherry tomatoes, cut in half

Bring a small pan of water to a boil, add the potatoes, and boil for 10–12 minutes until just cooked. Trim the beans, cut in half, and add to the potatoes 2 minutes before the end of cooking time. Drain.

Mix together the pesto and olive oil in a large bowl, add the potatoes and beans, and the tuna and tomatoes. Mix everything together, let cool, and store in the fridge until needed.

My niece Clare often makes Red Pasta Salad for her lunch. It is a great recipe for using up leftover sausages. If you need to cook some sausages, try the sesame and honey recipe on page 73. Vary the type of pasta you use since little changes help to keep things more interesting for your child. Use wholewheat pasta as often as possible, because it provides slow-release energy and fiber. I have used chipolata sausages, simply because they are thin and slice into good, bite-size pieces. I have suggested that this recipe serves 2, so you can have some for your lunch, too.

Jasmin, my middle daughter, thinks Tuna & Corn Pasta is the best packed lunch recipe ever! As with so many of the lunch ideas in this book, you can use this recipe as a guide and mix and match the ingredients.

**great variation** Salmon and Pea Pasta is a tasty alternative to the Tuna and Corn Pasta. Make the recipe as per the Tuna and Corn Pasta, but use canned salmon instead of tuna and cook some frozen or fresh peas instead of the corn.

# pasta salads

### red pasta salad

**serves** 2

1½ cups amori pasta shapes (or any of your choice)

3–4 teaspoons red pesto

4 teaspoons sour cream or crème fraîche (if available)

2 chipolata sausages, cooked according to package instructions and cooled

½ red bell pepper, seeded and chopped

6 cherry tomatoes, finely chopped

Bring a pot of water to a boil, add the pasta, and cook according to the instructions on the package. Drain and return to the pot.

In a small bowl, mix together the red pesto and sour cream.

Thinly slice the cooled sausages diagonally. Add the pepper, tomatoes, and sausages to the pasta and tip in the pesto mixture. Mix everything together, let cool, and store in the fridge until needed.

### tuna & corn pasta

**serves** 2

1½ cups pasta spirals or penne (or any of your choice)

1 x 6¼-oz. can tuna in sunflower oil, drained

7 oz. canned corn, drained and rinsed, (or cook about 1⅓–1½ cups frozen or fresh corn)

1 tablespoon mayonnaise

1 tablespoon plain yogurt

freshly ground black pepper

Bring a large pot of water to a boil, add the pasta, and cook according to the instructions on the package. Drain, put into a bowl, and let cool.

Add the tuna and corn.

Mix together the mayonnaise and yogurt with a little black pepper. Add the mayonnaise mixture to the pasta and mix together. Store in the fridge, ready to serve.

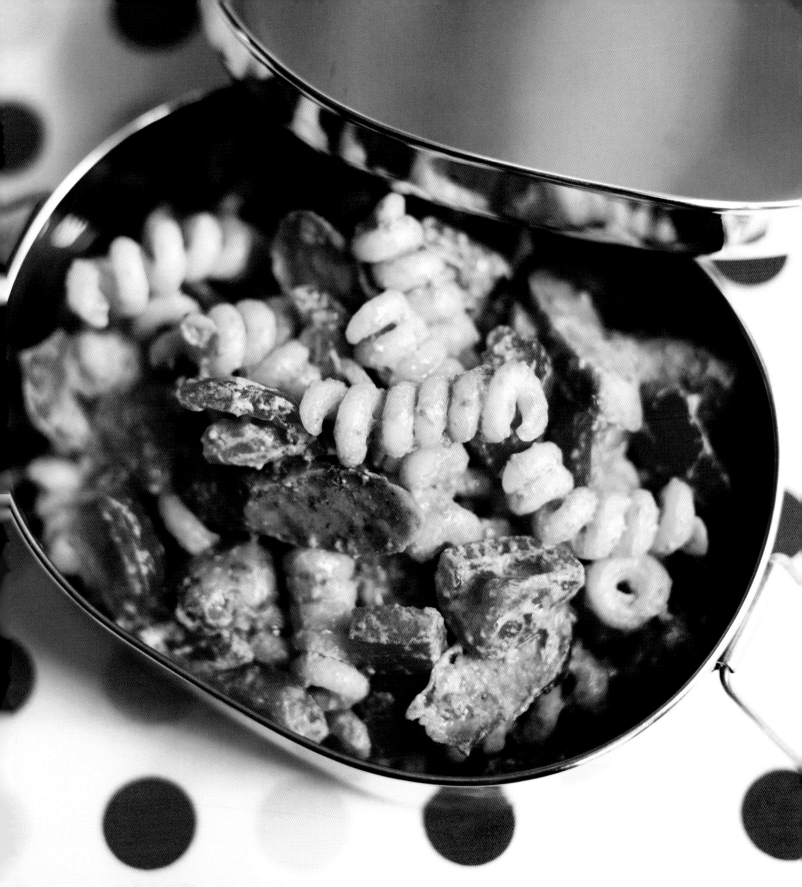

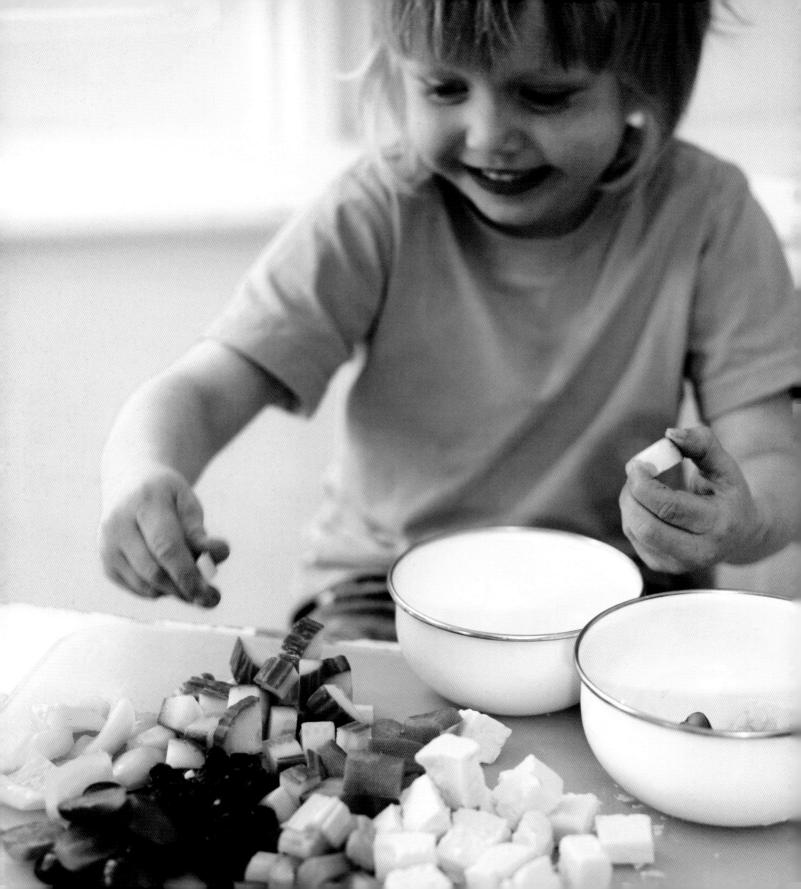

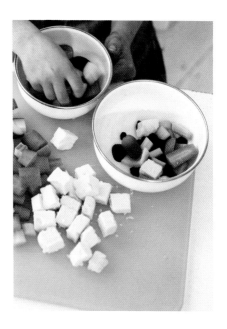

# pick 'n' mix salad

Although this seems like a very simple recipe, it is important to encourage children to enjoy eating fresh vegetables, like cucumber, celery, and carrots, which is why I have included this idea in my book. Given half the chance, my eldest daughter would choose to have Pick 'n' Mix Salad most days. Let your child help you decide what you put into the pick 'n' mix bowl.

Put all the vegetables into a bowl, and add the grapes, cheese, and raisins. Store in the fridge, ready to serve. This is best eaten with fingers. Pack a soft roll, some plain crackers, or rice cakes with this salad to make a quick and easy lunch.

**serves** 2

¼ cucumber, cut into bite-size chunks

2 stalks celery, cut into bite-size chunks

2 carrots, peeled and cut into sticks

a handful of red grapes

a small piece of cheddar (approximately 1-inch square), cut into bite-size chunks

a handful of raisins

2 soft rolls, for serving

One small cabbage will make enough for about 4 portions of coleslaw. You may need to keep trying this recipe if your child turns his/her nose up the first time you give it to them.

You can be as creative with this recipe as you like—try adding grated apple (doused in lemon juice to stop it from going brown), beet, celery, or red cabbage. Serve the vegetables thinly sliced so it's easier for children to eat and more appealing.

# coleslaw

Cut the cabbage into quarters, cut out the hard core, and then thinly slice the cabbage and put it into a bowl.

Add the carrots and pepper to the cabbage along with the raisins. Add peanuts if you like.

In a small bowl, mix together the mayonnaise yogurt, and honey and season with a little black pepper. Add to the coleslaw and mix well. Store in the fridge, ready to serve.

**nutrition tip** If your child does not like eating cooked cabbage, making coleslaw is a good way of sneaking it into his/her diet.

**serves 4**

1 small head or ½ large white or green cabbage

2 carrots, peeled and grated

1 red bell pepper, seeded and thinly sliced

a large handful of raisins

a large handful of peanuts (optional)

2 tablespoons mayonnaise or salad dressing

1 tablespoon plain yogurt

1 tablespoon honey

freshly ground black pepper

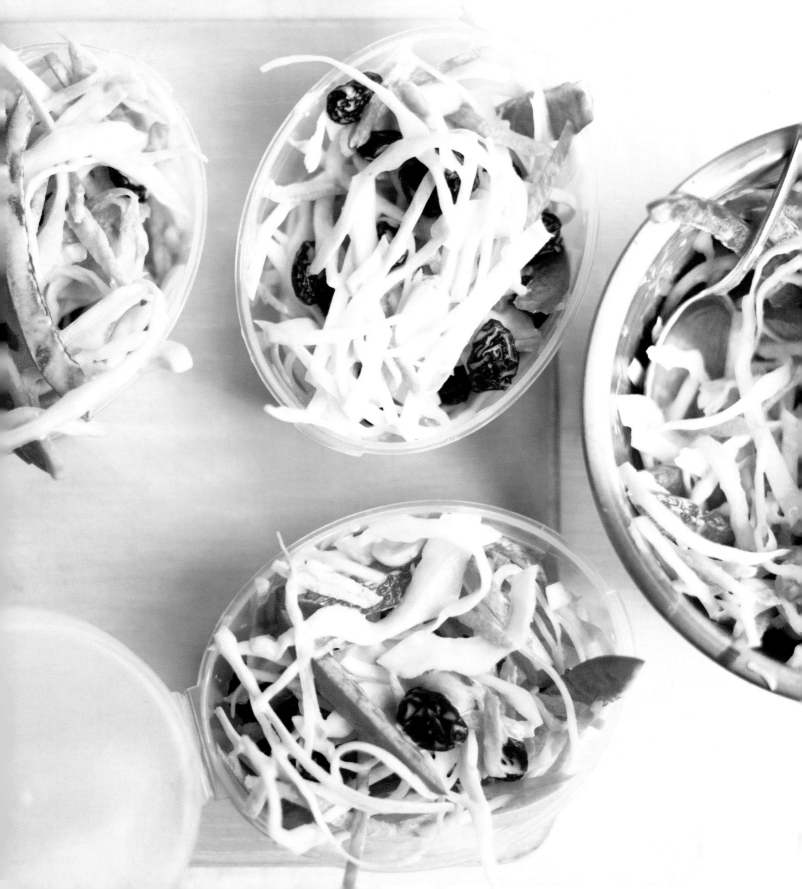

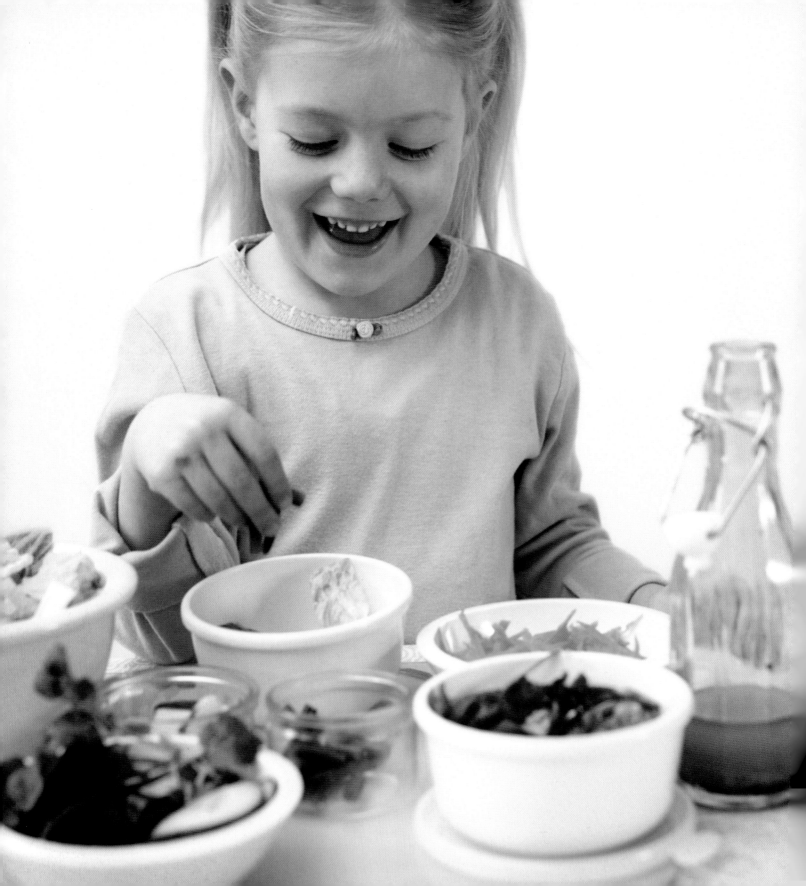

Many parents tell me that they just can't persuade their children to eat salad. One of the first pieces of advice I give them is to let their child make a dressing. Once children begin to mix and blend oils with vinegar or lemon juice, and honey or garlic, they become quite excited about drizzling this over their greens.

You shouldn't think of green salads as boring—children can actually find the different textures and flavors quite interesting. From experience, the key to success is to make sure that the salad is interesting to look at and easy to eat (everything should be cut into small pieces).

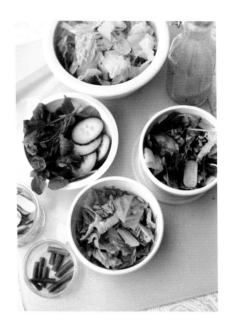

# green salad

**serves 2**

2 handfuls of crunchy lettuce leaves, washed and cut into small pieces

2 handfuls of baby spinach leaves or watercress, washed

**optional extras**

a small chunk of cucumber, thinly sliced

a large handful of green beans, trimmed and blanched

2 radishes (some children like the spiciness of these)

beet, sliced

carrot, peeled and grated

a large handful of seeds and nuts

**dressing**

3 tablespoons extra virgin olive oil

½–1 tablespoon lemon juice, or white or red wine vinegar, or balsamic vinegar

**with any of these:**

1 tablespoon honey

½ small garlic clove, crushed

½ teaspoon prepared mustard

Put the lettuce and baby spinach into a pot with a selection of the optional extras and mix together.

Make the dressing by mixing together the olive oil and lemon juice, and add more flavor with honey, garlic, or mustard, if you like.

Pack the dressing separately in a small jar or pot, so your child can drizzle this onto the salad before eating. This will prevent the leaves from wilting.

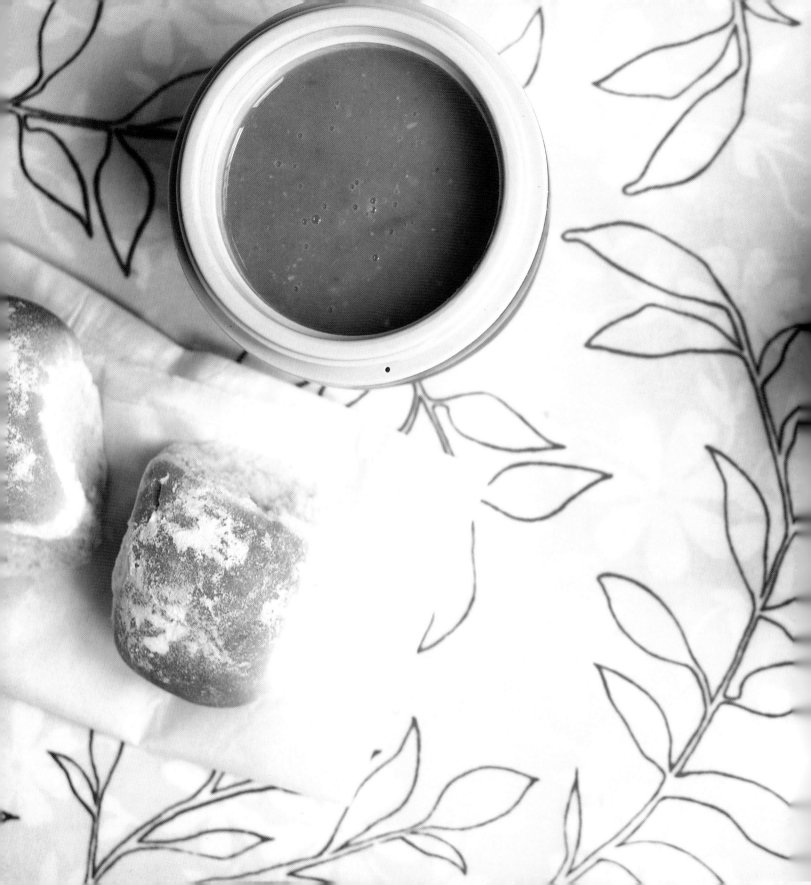

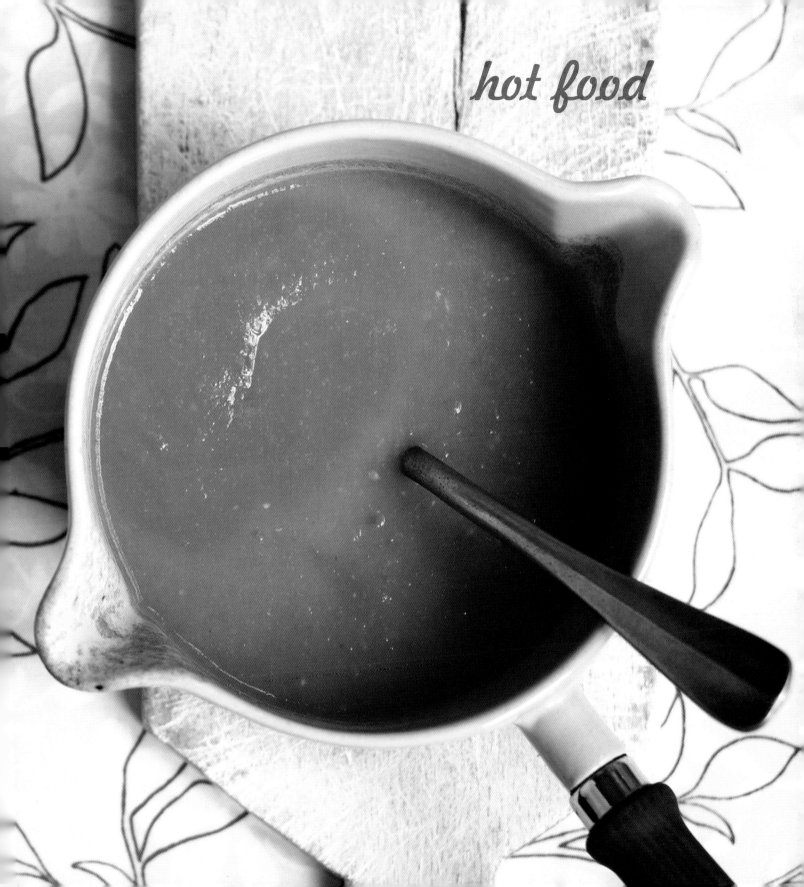

You can make this recipe for an evening meal and then keep enough for a packed lunch the next day. Make sure you heat it through before you put it into the thermos. Feel free to vary this recipe according to what you have in stock.

# chicken & red bell pepper stew

2 tablespoons olive oil

8 boneless chicken thighs

2 onions, finely chopped

1 garlic clove, peeled and crushed

2 red bell peppers, seeded and cut into bite-size pieces

1¼ cups chicken or vegetable broth

1½ cups canned cannellini beans, drained and rinsed

freshly ground black pepper

a pinch of light brown sugar (optional)

**serves 4**

*a heavy ovenproof pan*

1  Preheat the oven to 350°F. Heat half the oil in a heavy ovenproof pan, fry the chicken thighs until lightly browned all over, and transfer to a plate.

2  Add the remaining oil to the pan, then add the onions, garlic, and red bell pepper, and fry gently for 10–15 minutes until very soft, but not brown.

3  Add the broth to the mixture in the pan and place in the oven for 1 hour.

4  Spoon half of the sauce from the pan into a blender and whiz until smooth. Put back into the pan.

5  Add the cannellini beans and chicken to the pan and cook for another 15 minutes until the chicken is cooked through. Cut the chicken into bite-size pieces.

6  Season with black pepper and a pinch of light soft brown sugar, if you think it is needed. Serve for dinner and set some aside to cool for your child's lunch the next day. Wait until it has fully cooled, put in an airtight container, and store in the fridge. Make sure you heat it through thoroughly before putting it in a thermos.

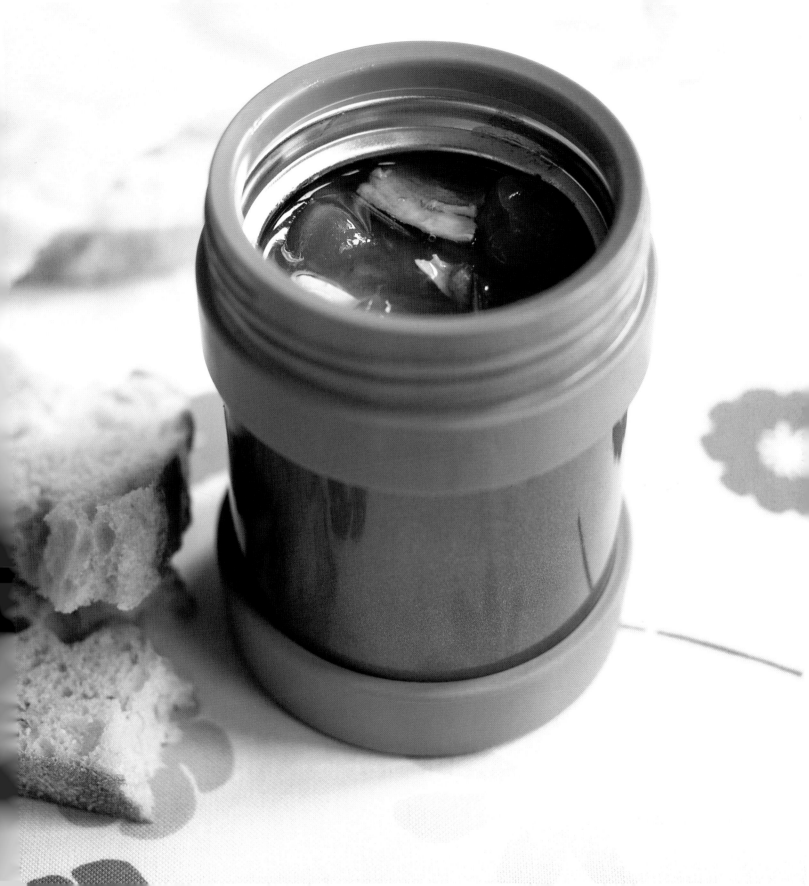

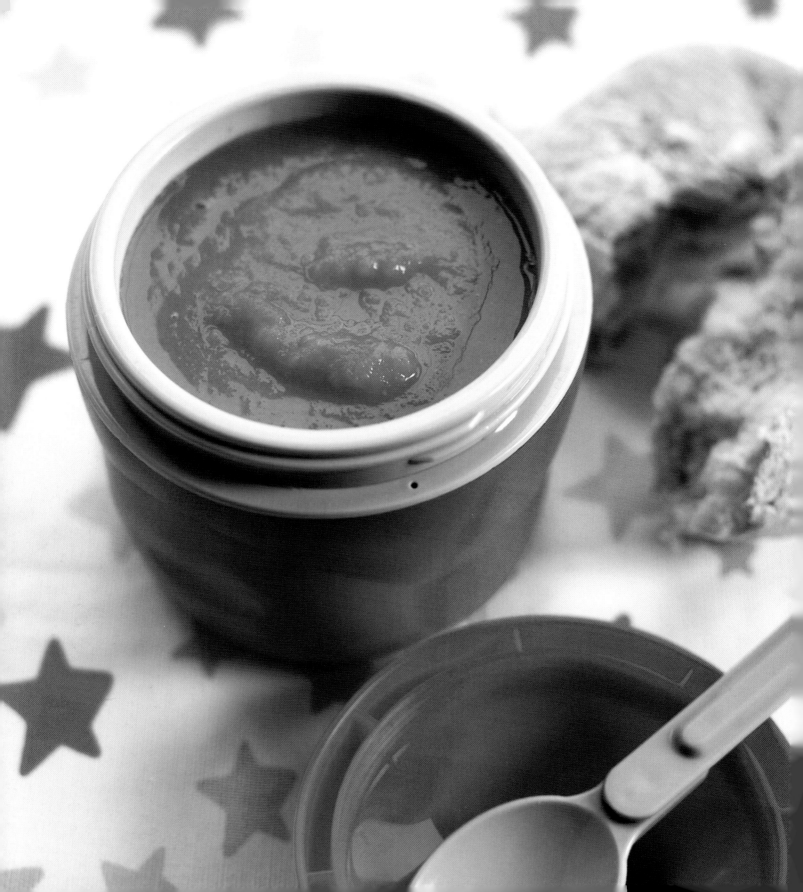

This is my basic recipe for tomato soup. The key to success is first to choose ripe tomatoes, and secondly to let them stew for a while so that they reduce to a mush (this will help give the tomatoes an intense flavor). Most children love a creamy tomato soup, especially if you give them a fresh roll that they can dunk in it.

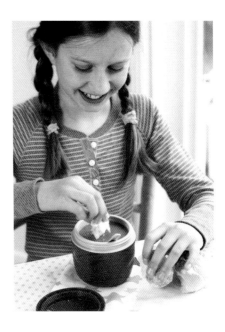

# tomato soup

**1** Heat the olive oil and butter in a saucepan, then fry the onion and garlic—this will take a good 10 minutes. You want them to soften, but not turn too brown. When the onion is soft, add the tomatoes and simmer gently, stirring occasionally until the tomatoes have turned to mush and most of the liquid has evaporated. This will take another 20 minutes.

**2** Add the broth, bring to a boil, reduce the heat and simmer gently for 15 minutes.

**3** Puree the soup in a blender or food processor. Return to the pan, warm it through, and add the sugar and black pepper.

**4** If you want to make this soup really creamy, add a little cream or milk. Serve with a soft roll.

1 tablespoon olive oil

a pat of butter

1 onion, peeled and finely chopped

1 garlic clove, finely chopped

12 ripe tomatoes, halved

3¼ cups light chicken or vegetable broth

a pinch of light brown sugar

freshly ground black pepper

a little cream (optional)

soft rolls, for dunking

**serves 4**

8 chipolata sausages

4 strips of bacon

2 tablespoons olive oil

1 garlic clove, peeled and crushed

1 x 14-oz. can chopped tomatoes

1¾ cups tomato puree

2–2½ cups chicken or vegetable broth (to achieve desired consistency)

15-oz. can chickpeas, drained and rinsed

1 teaspoon light brown sugar (optional)

a handful of fresh thyme leaves, chopped

freshly ground black pepper

**serves 4**

If you are making this for a meal at home, you could also try adding some thinly sliced cabbage just before the end of cooking, but if it is going to later be taken to school in a thermos, it's best to leave the cabbage out as it tends to go soggy with time.

If your child likes spicy food, try using chorizo sausage instead of chipolatas. Make sure that you keep all the pieces small, so that it is easy to eat.

# sausage & bean casserole

1  Preheat the oven to 350°F.

2  Roast the sausages for 25–30 minutes, turning occasionally until cooked through and golden. Slice diagonally into bite-size pieces. Set to one side.

3  Snip the bacon into small pieces using a pair of scissors.

4  Heat the oil in a large heavy saucepan and fry the bacon until golden. Add the garlic and cook for 1 minute. Add the tomatoes, tomato puree, broth, chickpeas, sausages, sugar, thyme, and black pepper to taste, and simmer for another 20–25 minutes.

5  Serve for dinner and set some aside to cool for your child's lunch the next day. Wait until it has fully cooled, then put in an airtight container and store in the fridge. Heat through thoroughly the next day before putting it in a thermos.

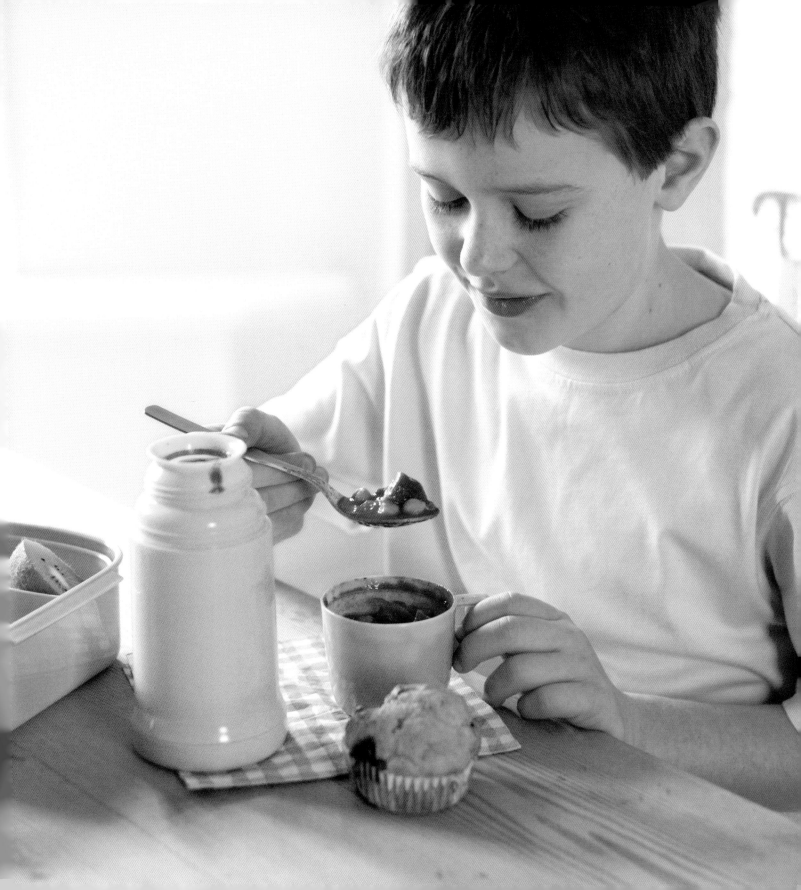

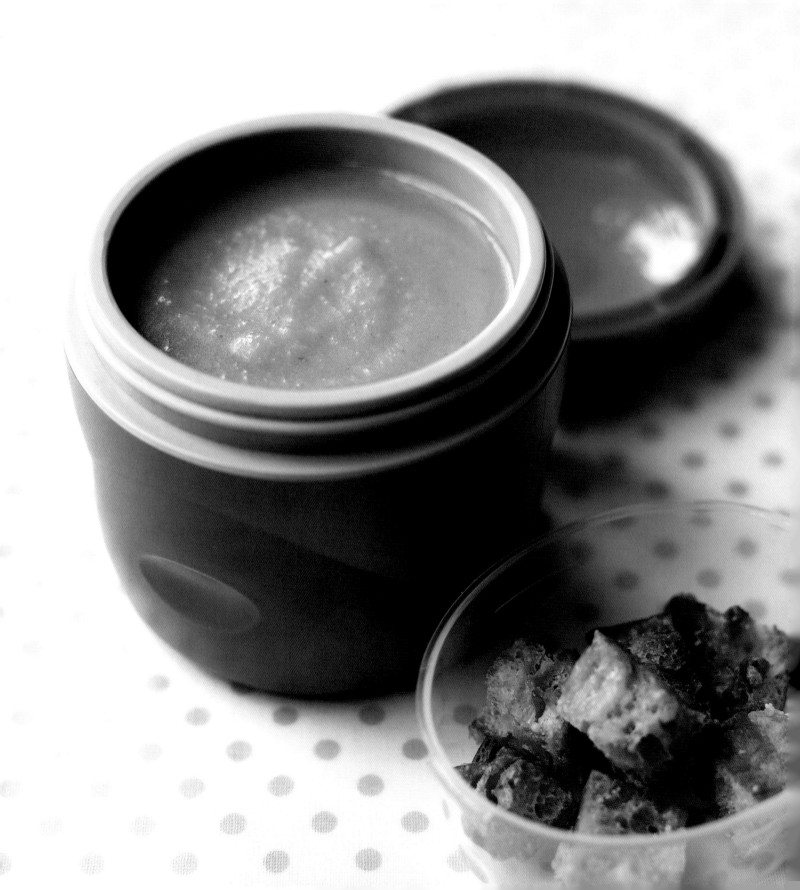

The hint of sweetness in this butternut squash soup makes it appealing to children. To keep things as easy and quick as possible, roast the vegetables to bring out their sweetness and then puree them to make the soup. Add enough broth to suit your child's taste—some children find soup easier to eat if it is thicker in texture.

# butternut squash soup

**1** Preheat the oven to 375°F.

**2** Cut the butternut squash in half, scoop out the seeds, and peel it—you will need to use a sharp knife to cut the tough skin away. Cut the flesh into big pieces.

**3** Put all the vegetables into a heavy roasting dish, add the garlic, and drizzle the oil over everything—you may want to use your hands to mix everything together. Roast for 30–40 minutes.

**4** Put the roasted vegetables into a food processor (squeeze the garlic out of the skins), with the broth—you may need to do this in two batches. Puree until smooth.

**5** Pour into a saucepan, and season to taste with black pepper and a little honey. Heat gently.

**For the Parmesan croutons:** For the croutons, reduce the oven temperature to 350°F. Put the diced bread cubes into a roasting tray, drizzle with the oil, and sprinkle with the Parmesan. Toss everything together. Put in the oven and roast for 5–10 minutes, turning occasionally, until light golden.

Put the croutons in a small airtight container or bag, so your child can add them to his/her soup at lunchtime. If you add them in the thermos, they will dissolve into the soup.

1 butternut squash (about 3 lbs)

2 onions, cut into thin wedges

3 carrots, peeled and cut into thirds, widthwise

2 stalks celery, cut in half

3 garlic cloves (unpeeled)

1 tablespoon olive oil

3–4 cups boiling vegetable broth

freshly ground black pepper

a little honey

Parmesan croutons

3 thick slices of bread, cubed

olive oil, for drizzling

Parmesan cheese, for sprinkling

serves 4

*a heavy roasting dish*

*a food processor*

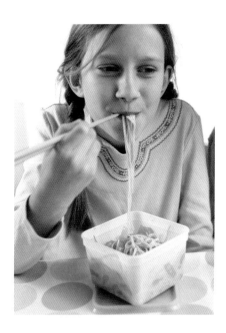

**nutrition tip** Pineapples contain vitamin C, which children need to help boost their immune system. They also contain potassium and an enzyme that breaks down protein, which helps digestion.

These noodles can be reheated the morning after you've made them and put in a thermos, so that they're nice and hot for your child at lunchtime. Alternatively, you can serve them cold in an airtight container.

# noodles

2 tablespoons red or white wine vinegar

¼ cup tomato paste

2 tablespoons light brown sugar

½ teaspoon mustard powder

1 teaspoon reduced salt soy sauce

4 bundles Chinese-style dried egg noodles or straight-to-wok noodles

2 teaspoons sunflower oil

2 teaspoons sesame oil

2 scallions, thinly sliced

1 small garlic clove, peeled and crushed

2 handfuls each of sugar snap peas, baby corn, sliced green bell peppers

14-/15-oz. can pineapple pieces in juice

**serves 4**

1 In a bowl, mix together the vinegar, tomato paste, sugar, mustard powder, and soy sauce. Set aside.

2 Bring a large pot of water to a boil and cook the noodles according to the package instructions. Drain and set aside.

3 Heat the oils in a skillet, add the scallions, garlic, and vegetables, and stir-fry for a few minutes—you want them to be cooked, but still crisp.

4 Add the vinegar mixture and cook for a few minutes. Add the pineapple pieces and juice and continue to cook for a few more minutes until the liquid has reduced. Add the noodles and toss everything together.

5 Set the noodles aside to cool and store in the fridge, ready to serve.

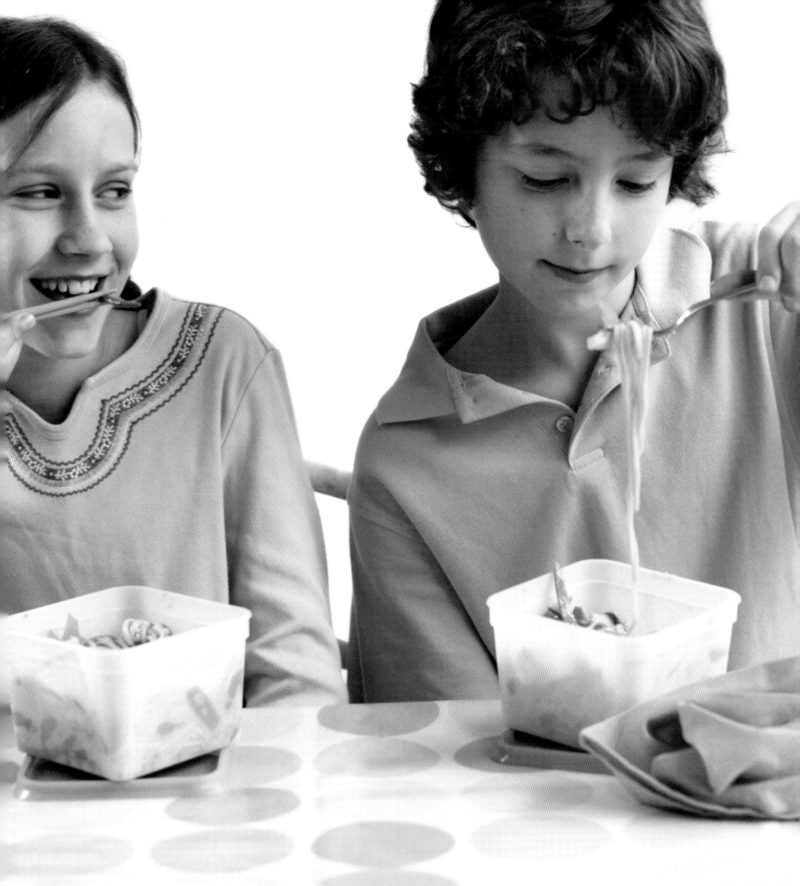

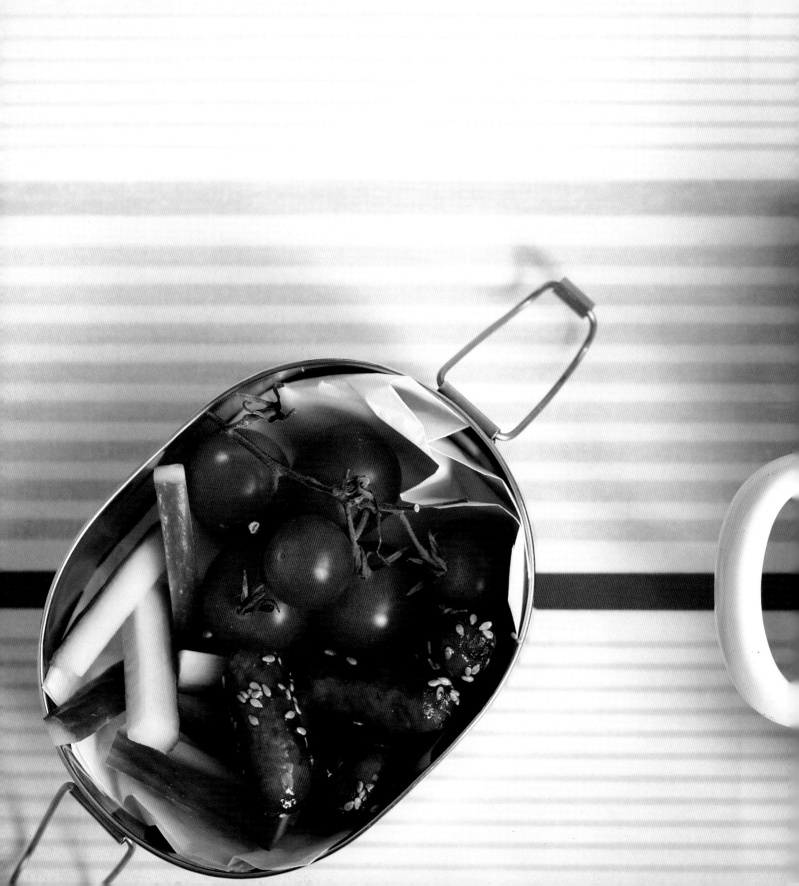

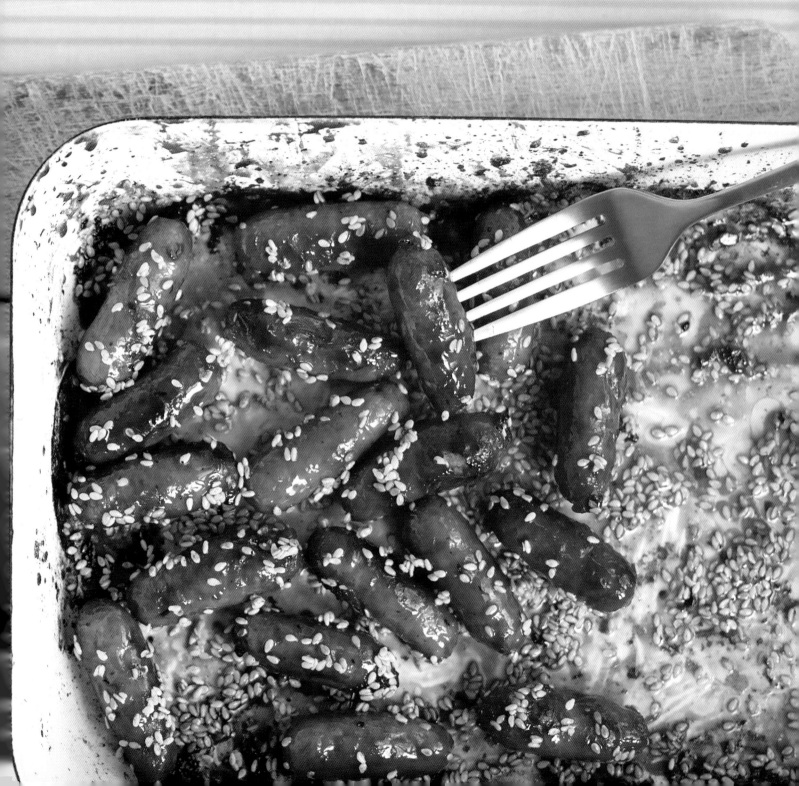

# cheese straws

This simple cheese pastry recipe is not only quick, but tasty. I tend to cut the straws into small lengths so that they don't break in the lunchbox. Depending on what you have available in your fridge, you can make the pastry with most cheeses—e.g. Swiss cheese or Parmesan. Get your children to make these—they will love rubbing the butter into the flour and rolling out the pastry.

a heaping cup all-purpose flour, plus extra for dusting

3 tablespoons butter, chilled and cut into small pieces, plus extra for greasing

⅓–½ cup strong cheddar, grated

1 small egg, beaten

**makes** approximately 12

*a baking sheet, greased*

1 Preheat the oven to 350°F.

2 Sift the flour into a large bowl. Rub the butter into the flour using your fingertips until the mixture looks like fine bread crumbs. Add the grated cheese and mix together.

3 Add the beaten egg and stir into the flour until the mixture starts to come together. Then use your hands to work it into a ball.

4 Sprinkle some flour onto the counter and onto a rolling pin. Roll out half the dough into a rectangle about ⅛-inch thick. Cut widthwise into straws. Carefully lift them onto the baking sheet, leaving a little space between each one. Bake for 10 minutes, until golden.

5 Let the straws cool for a couple of minutes on the baking sheet and then carefully transfer them to a wire rack. Eat warm or let cool completely and store in an airtight container.

# pesto cheese twists

This is a quick alternative to the Cheese Straws recipe. You can try these with grainy mustard instead of the pesto if your child fancies something a little different. They are also suitable for freezing, so ideal for popping in your child's lunchbox as a quick fuss-free snack.

a little butter, for greasing

all-purpose flour, for dusting

13-oz. (1½ sheets from a 490 g package) ready-rolled puff pastry dough (thawed if frozen)

about ¾–1 cup cheese, grated, e.g. cheddar, Parmesan

2–3 tablespoons pesto or grainy mustard

**makes** 30

*2 baking sheets, greased*

1 Preheat the oven to 400°F.

2 Sprinkle the counter with a little flour and spread out the pastry dough.

3 Sprinkle the cheese evenly over half the dough, then fold it in half. Using a rolling pin, roll the dough back out to its original size.

4 Using a pastry spatula or butter knife, spread the pesto over half of the dough and fold in half. Roll it back out to its original size. Cut into long thin straws.

5 Hold the end of a straw in one hand. Use your other hand to turn the other end of the straw to create a twisted shape. Lay it on a baking sheet. Repeat with the other straws, leaving a little space between each one on the baking sheets.

6 Bake for 8–10 minutes.

7 Remove from the oven, carefully lift the straws off the baking sheet and put them onto a wire rack. Eat them warm or else let cool completely and store in an airtight container.

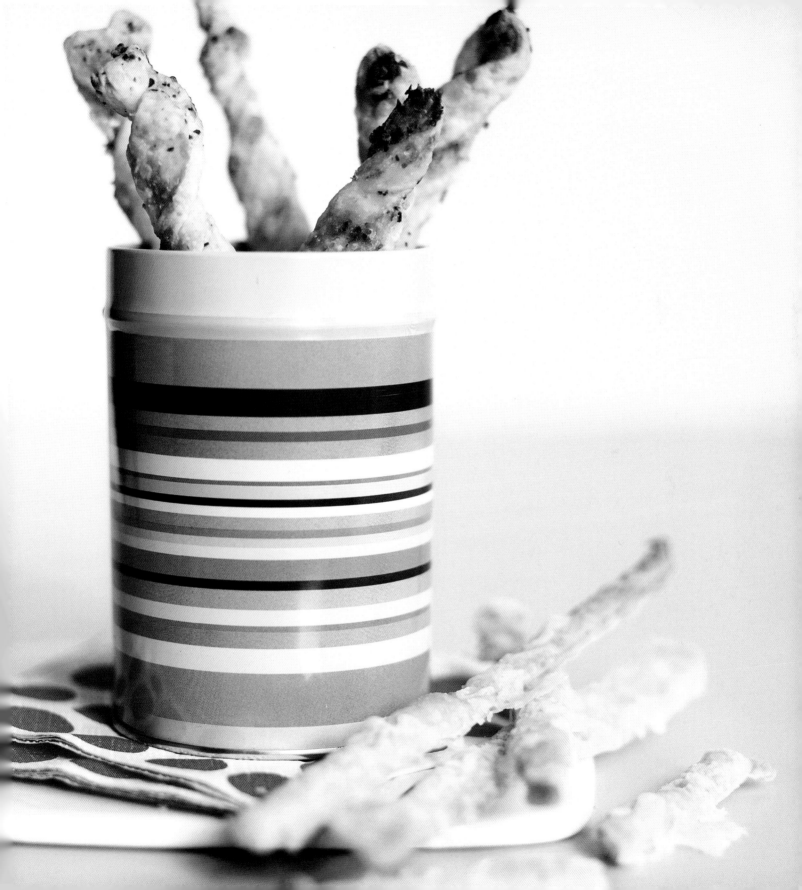

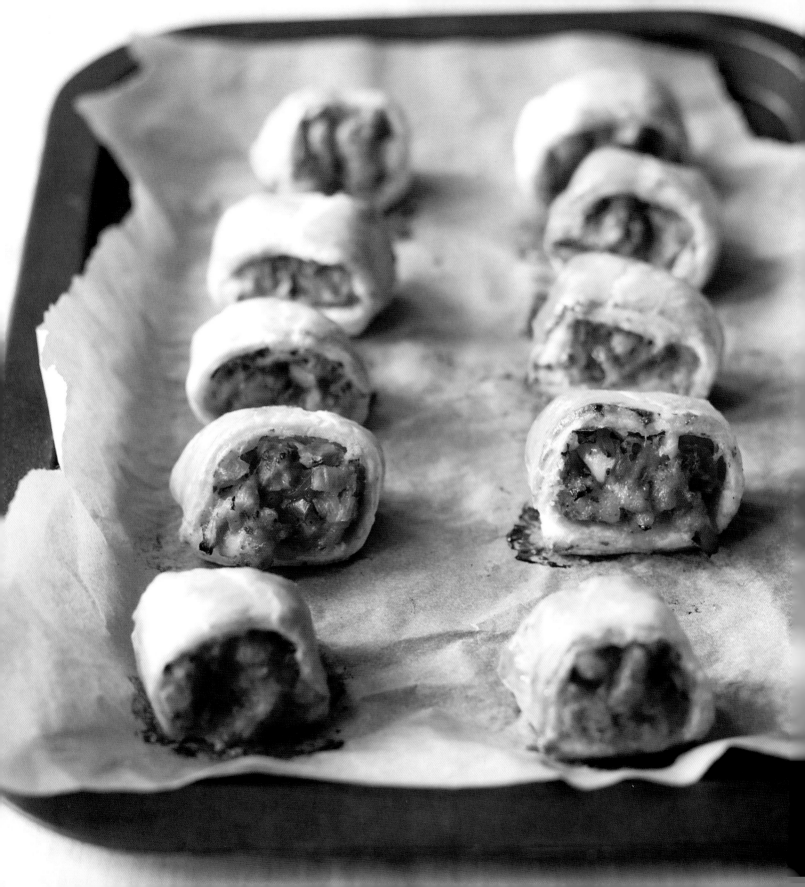

Red bell peppers contain fantastic vitamins, like betacarotene and vitamin C—both essential for helping to boost immature immune systems. Try as often as possible to add vegetables to your child's favorite foods.

# sausage & red pepper rolls

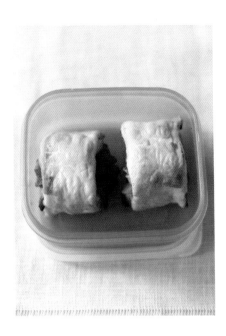

1. Preheat the oven to 400°F.

2. Dust your counter with a little flour and roll out the pastry dough until it is approximately 12 x 11 inches and then cut in half lengthwise.

3. Heat the oil in a skillet, add the onion and pepper, and sauté for 5 minutes or until soft. Add the chopped apple and cook for 1 minute. Let cool slightly.

4. Put the sausage meat into a bowl, add the onion mixture and parsley (if using), and season with a little freshly ground black pepper and mix together.

5. Divide the sausage meat mixture into two equal halves and shape each into a long sausage shape. Place each sausage shape along the long edge of each piece of pastry dough. Brush the opposite edge of the dough with beaten egg and roll up from the sausage edge. Seal the pastry edges and turn the rolls over so that the seam is underneath.

6. Cut each roll into 1-inch lengths. Cut a small slit in the top of each roll, brush with beaten egg, and pop onto the baking sheets. Bake for 20–25 minutes. Remove from the oven, transfer to a wire rack, and let cool.

all-purpose flour, for dusting

13-oz (1½ sheets from a 490 g package) ready-rolled puff pastry dough (thawed if frozen)

1 tablespoon olive oil

1 onion, finely chopped

1 red bell pepper, seeded and finely chopped

1 apple, cored and finely chopped

1 lb good-quality bulk pork sausage

1 handful fresh parsley, chopped (optional)

freshly ground black pepper

1 egg, beaten

**makes 18–20**

**alternative filling**

1 lb ground chicken,
1 tablespoon honey, and
2 teaspoons whole-grain mustard

2 *large baking sheets, greased*

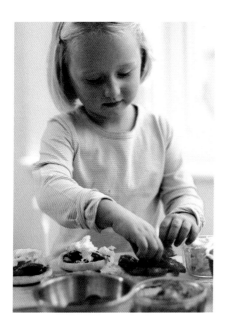

If your child likes cold pizza, why not make one to pop into his/her lunchbox? You can make these pizzas with rolls, muffins, or French baguettes. Prepare these pizzas the night before—cook one for the lunchbox, and keep the other in the fridge until you need it for your own lunch.

# easy pizzas

2 English muffins or 1 thin part-baked French baguette

1 garlic clove

2–3 tablespoons tomato paste

**toppings**

salami, ham (shredded), canned tuna in sunflower oil (drained), corn (drained), thinly sliced red bell pepper (seeded), green or black olives (pitted and cut in half)

2 handfuls of grated cheddar

6 slices mozzarella (optional)

**serves** 2

**1** Preheat the oven to 375°F.

**2** Cut the muffin in half lengthwise and lightly toast each half. Rub the cut side of each half with the garlic.

**3** Spread the tomato paste over the muffin. Top with your child's favorite toppings, sprinkle with the cheddar, and lay the mozzarella on top, if using.

**4** Cook in the oven for 5–8 minutes until golden and bubbling. Let cool.

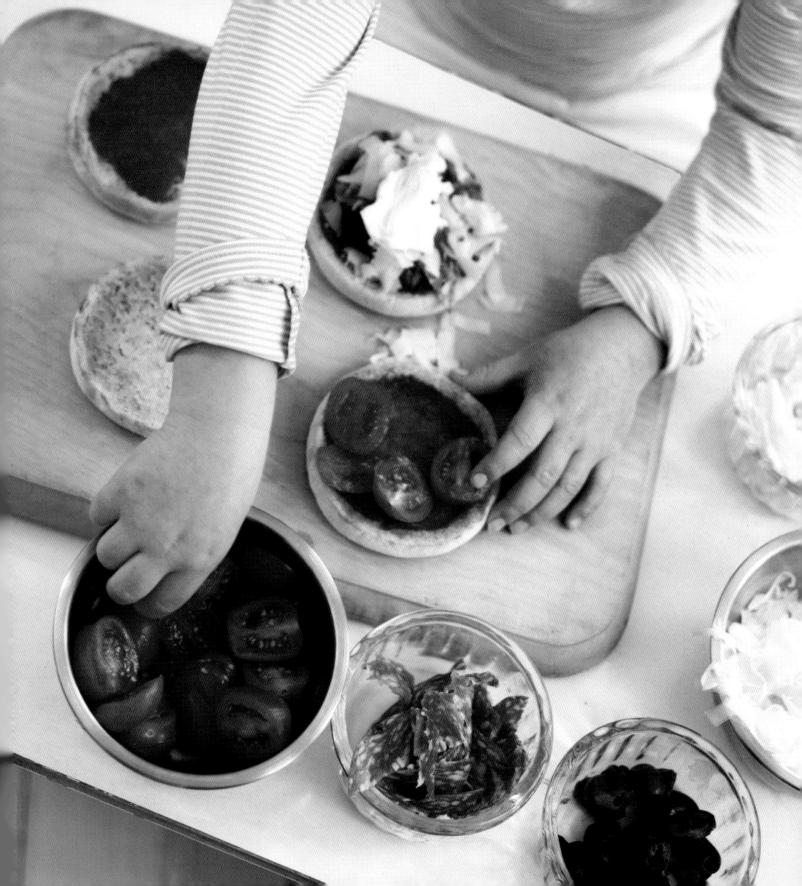

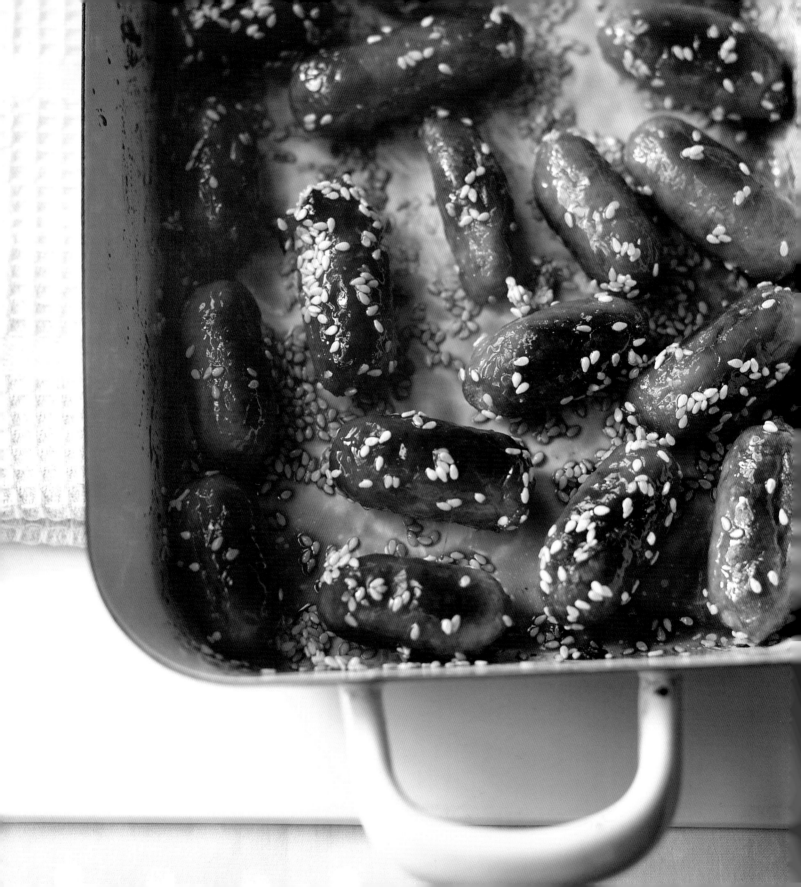

This is a quick recipe idea for sausages—great for lunchboxes, but also a big hit at children's parties. You'll find that adults love these just as much as children do.

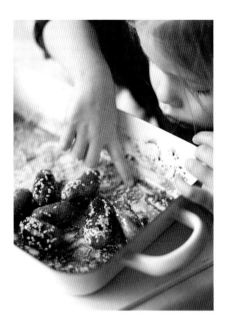

# sesame sausages

**1** Preheat the oven to 400°F. Twist the sausages in the middle and then cut in half.

**2** Scatter the sausages in a roasting dish and cook for 15–20 minutes, turning once. Drain off any fat. Add the honey and cook for another 15 minutes, turning a couple of times until the sausages are sticky and golden all over.

**3** Sprinkle the sesame seeds over the sausages and cook for 5 minutes longer. Serve hot or cold.

12 good-quality chipolatas

2 tablespoons honey

2 tablespoons sesame seeds

*a heavy-based roasting dish*

**serves** 4

**nutrition tip** Most children need small snacks in between meals to help prevent blood sugar and energy lows. Fresh fruits or vegetables are ideal snacks, but for those times when your child's craving something a little bit more filling, a small sesame sausage can fill the gap.

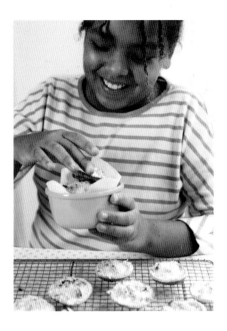

Make these in the evening or at the weekend, when things are not quite so manic. Ask the children to help you to make the dough—they love to rub the butter into the flour and roll and cut out the shapes. Alternatively, buy some puff pastry dough and use this instead. Vary the fillings—try tuna and corn, chopped cooked bacon and cheese, and broccoli and salmon. Equally, if you don't have any heavy cream in your fridge, use another egg and a little more milk.

# mini quiches

**for the pastry dough:**

1⅔ cups all-purpose flour, plus extra for dusting

½ cup (1 stick) butter, chilled and cut into small pieces

1 egg yolk

**for the filling:** 1 small onion, finely chopped (or 3 scallions, finely chopped)

1 small garlic clove, crushed (optional)

1 tablespoon olive oil

1 egg, beaten

⅓ cup heavy cream

⅓ cup milk

2 skinless salmon fillets, cut into small cubes

a couple of handfuls finely grated Parmesan

**makes 18**

*an 18-cup muffin pan, greased*

1. Preheat the oven to 400°F.

2. Sift the flour into a large mixing bowl, add the butter and egg, and rub it in using your fingertips until the mixture looks like fine bread crumbs.

3. Add 1–2 tablespoons water, a little at a time, stirring until the mixture comes together as a ball. Cover and chill for 30 minutes.

4. Sprinkle the counter and your rolling pin with a little flour and roll the dough out to about ⅛-inch thick. Cut out circles to fit your muffin pan. Lay them in the muffin pan holes and prick the bottom of each mini-quiche crust once with a fork.

5. Bake for 5 minutes until the crust is a very pale golden color. Remove from the oven and set aside. Gently fry the onion and garlic in the oil until soft.

6. In a jug, mix together the egg, cream, and milk. Divide the onion mixture and salmon between each crust. Drizzle the egg mixture into each crust, sprinkle with the Parmesan, and bake for 5–6 minutes until risen, slightly golden, and set.

7. Remove from the oven and let cool for a few minutes before taking them out of the pan.

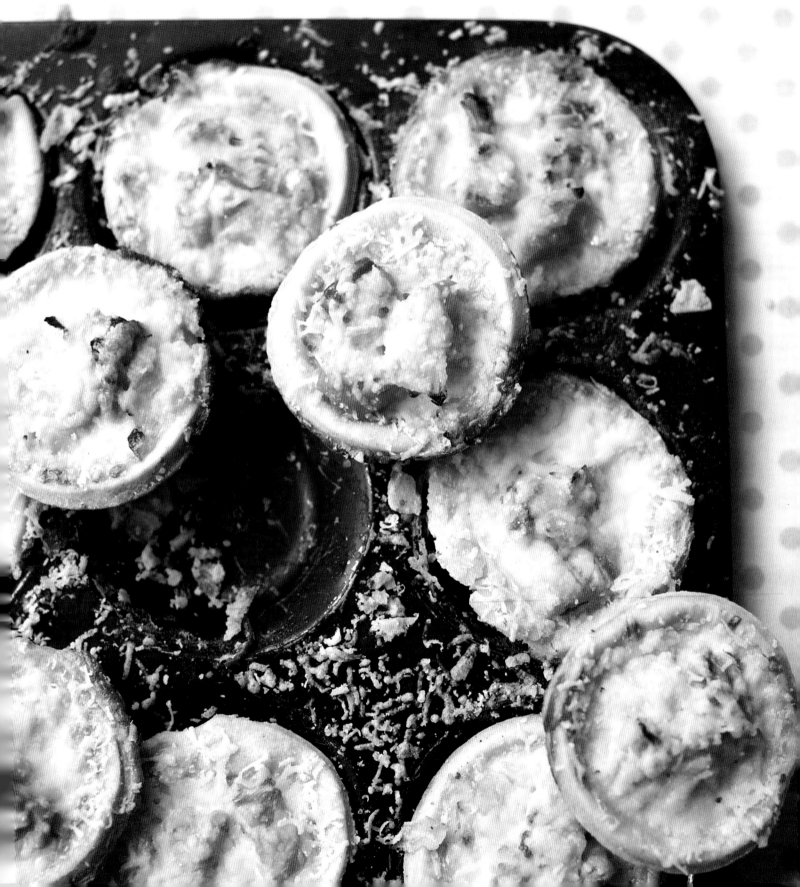

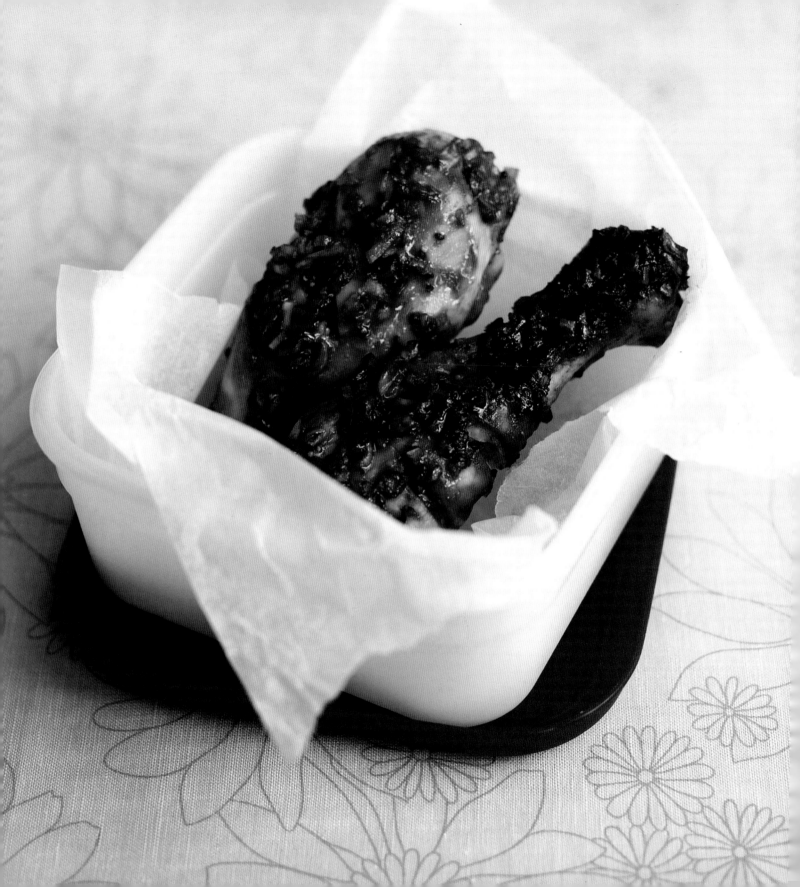

Cook these for supper and keep a couple in the fridge overnight ready for your child's lunchbox in the morning. Most children will enjoy nibbling the chicken off the bone, but if your child eats slowly, you might like to cut the chicken off the bone and pack it in a carton with a fork.

# chicken drumsticks

1. Preheat the oven to 400°F.

2. Score each piece of chicken with a knife about 2 or 3 times.

3. Put the onion into a large bowl, add all the other ingredients, and mix well.

4. Add the chicken and stir really well until each piece of chicken is covered—you may prefer to use your hands to really work the marinade into the chicken. Cover and chill for 15–30 minutes.

5. Put the chicken into a heavy baking dish and roast for 40–45 minutes. You may need to turn the chicken occasionally.

6. Let cool and keep in the fridge overnight, ready to pack in your child's lunchbox the next day.

8 chicken pieces (e.g., thighs, legs), skin removed

1 onion, peeled and finely chopped

½ cup tomato ketchup

2 tablespoons dark brown sugar

1 tablespoon whole-grain mustard

1 tablespoon Worcestershire sauce

1 garlic clove, crushed

**makes** 4 (2 chicken pieces per serving)

*a heavy baking dish*

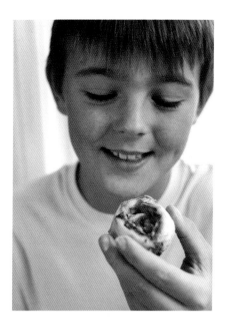

My middle daughter has never really enjoyed eating sandwiches, unless they are cut very small and are easy to eat. She much prefers these puff pastry pinwheels. I have experimented with a whole variety of fillings, but this combination has been incredibly popular with children. If you don't have pesto in your cupboard, you can try them without.

# puff pinwheels

4 strips of bacon

1 tablespoon olive oil

2 scallions, finely chopped

13-oz. (1½ sheets from a 490 g package) ready-rolled puff pastry dough (thawed if frozen)

2–3 tablespoons red pesto

1 cup grated cheddar

makes 20

*a baking sheet, greased*

**great variation** Tuna and Corn Mini Cornish Pasties. Mix together a 6–6¼-oz. can tuna, 2 handfuls cooked corn, and a little mayonnaise. Cut out approximately 20 circles from 1½ sheets of 490 g ready-rolled puff pastry dough. Fill half the circle with the tuna mixture. Fold the remaining half of the dough circle over the mixture and pinch the edges together to form a closed pocket. Place on a baking sheet and bake in the oven at 375°F until golden and cooked.

**1** Preheat the oven to 375°F.

**2** Cut the bacon into small pieces. Heat the oil in a skillet and fry the bacon for 4–8 minutes, until cooked. Add the scallions and cook gently until they are soft. Let cool slightly.

**3** Unroll the pastry dough sheets, spread with the red pesto and scatter over the bacon and scallions. Top with the grated cheddar. Carefully roll the dough, starting with a long side so that you end up with a long, thin sausage shape.

**4** Cut the sausage shape into 20 round pieces and place on a baking sheet. Bake for 10–12 minutes until golden and risen. Remove from the oven and let cool on a wire rack.

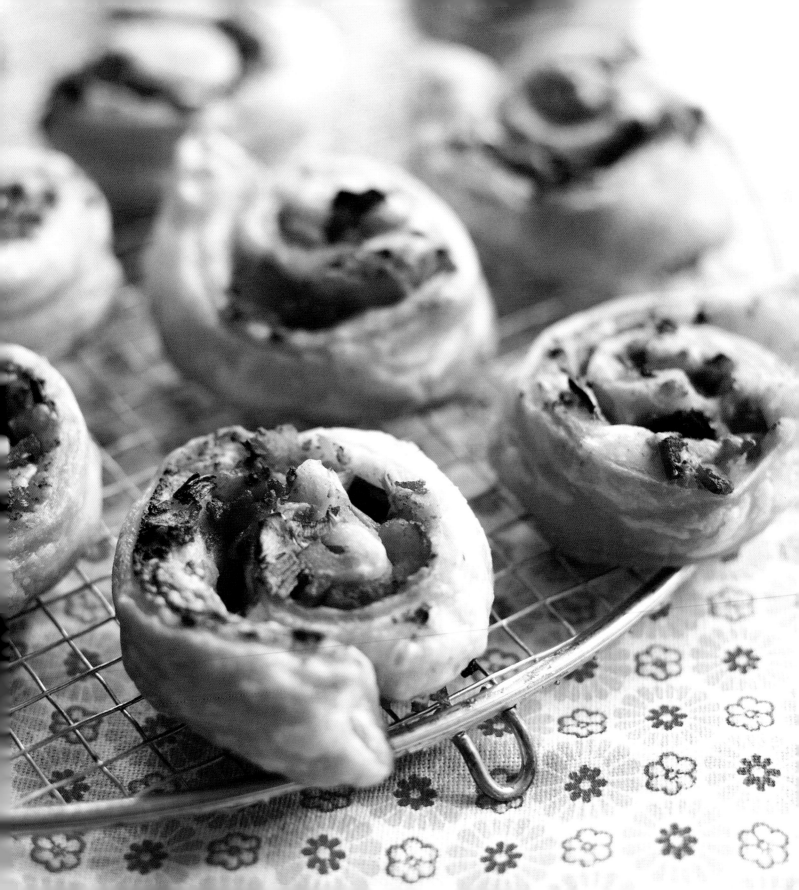

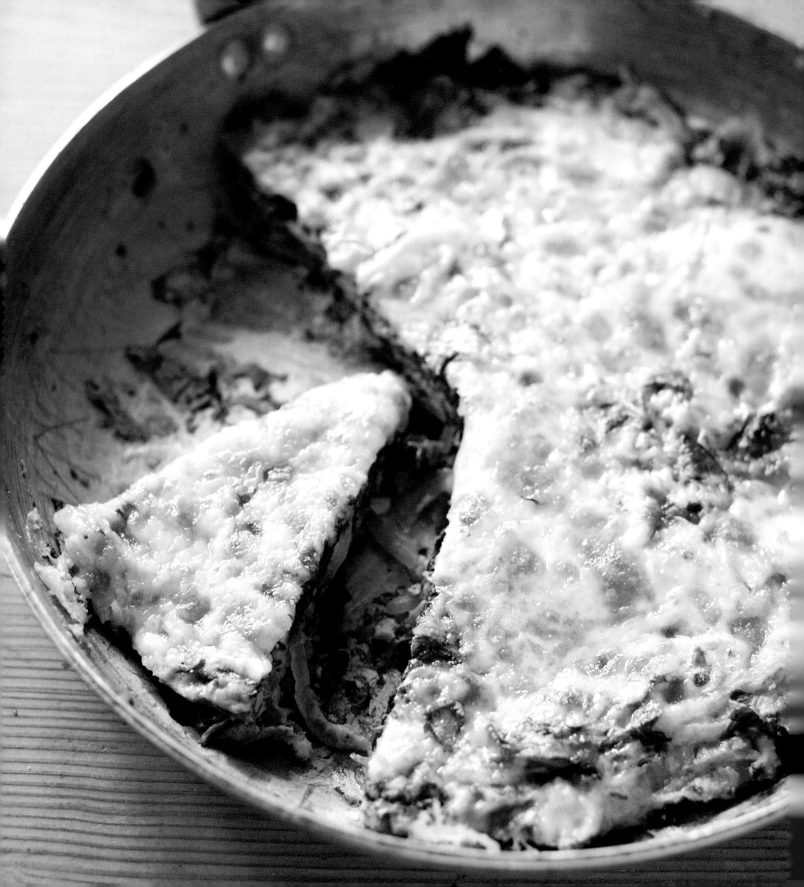

Leafy green vegetables, like spinach, contain omega-3, an important fatty acid that's known to help concentration. Spinach is also a good source of potassium, calcium, and iron. Chop it up and add to omelets, pasta sauces, or fish pies—an effective way of getting your child to eat greens.

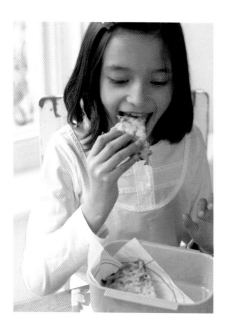

# spinach & onion tortilla

**1** Preheat the broiler to high.

**2** Break the eggs into a large bowl, season with salt and pepper, and beat briefly with a fork.

**3** Heat the oil in a large skillet with a heatproof handle and fry the onion until soft and pale golden. Add the spinach and sauté for a couple of minutes to wilt the leaves.

**4** Pour the egg mixture into the pan, turn the heat down to its lowest setting, and cook the tortilla, uncovered, for approximately 8 minutes, until there is only a little runny egg left on the top.

**5** Sprinkle the grated cheese over the top and place under the preheated broiler for 1–2 minutes, until the top is golden and bubbling.

**6** Use a spatula to slide the tortilla out onto a plate. Cut into wedges. Let cool and store in the fridge, ready to serve.

5 eggs, beaten

sea salt or kosher salt, and freshly ground black pepper

2 tablespoons olive oil

1 large Spanish onion, cut in half and thinly sliced

6 oz. (about 3 cups) fresh spinach leaves, washed and chopped

⅓–½ cup grated cheddar

**serves 4**

Mackerel has the highest omega-3 content of all oily fish. Children need omega-3 for healthy brain function. Oily fish, like other fish, also contains essential minerals and protein and is a good source of vitamin D. You can serve this as a lunchbox snack in a couple of different ways. It can be used as a dip and eaten with vegetable sticks or with strips of toast, used to fill pita breads or rolls, or spread onto soft tortillas and rolled up.

3 smoked mackerel fillets

½ cup plain yogurt

1 garlic clove, peeled and roughly chopped

1 tablespoon whole-grain mustard or 1–2 tablespoons horseradish (optional)

freshly squeezed juice of ½ lemon

freshly ground black pepper

strips of toast or vegetable sticks, for serving

**makes** 4 small tubs

*a food processor*

**nutrition tip** Mackerel is a great source of omega-3 essential fatty acids, which are associated with good brain development and mental health.

# smoked mackerel pâté

1 Remove the skin from the mackerel fillets and flake the fish into a food processor (or blender).

2 Add the yogurt, garlic, mustard, and lemon juice and puree until smooth. Season with a little freshly ground black pepper, if you like.

3 Put the dip into small airtight tubs and store in the fridge, ready to serve. Cut up some vegetable sticks or strips of toast to serve as an accompaniment. Store in the fridge and keep covered. It will keep for 2–3 days.

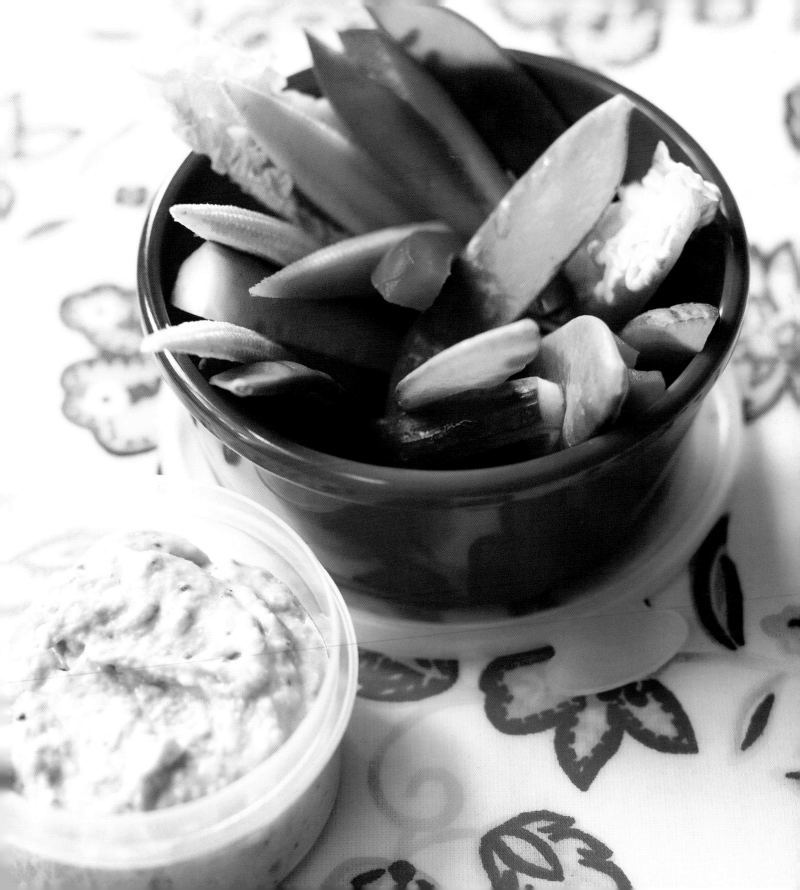

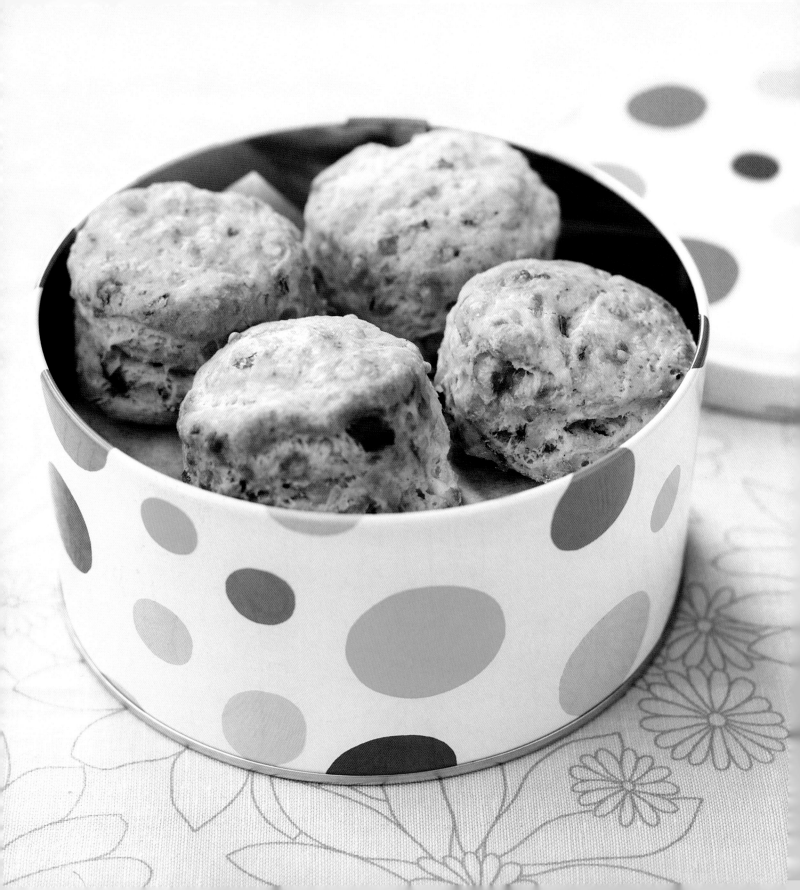

These scones are a great alternative to sandwiches—add some carrot or cucumber sticks and away you go! Make a batch and keep them in the freezer—put a frozen scone in your child's lunchbox in the morning and it will have thawed by lunchtime.

# pick 'n' mix scones

1 Preheat the oven to 400°F.

2 Sift the flour and baking powder into a large bowl. Add the butter and rub in until the mixture starts to look like fine bread crumbs.

3 Add a handful each of 2 fillings of your choice. Use a butter knife to mix in the milk, a little at a time (you may not need to add all of the milk), until the mixture starts to come together.

4 Sprinkle a little flour onto your counter, then tip the dough out of the bowl. Put a little flour on your hands and very lightly knead the mixture for ½ minute until it is smooth.

5 Form the mixture into a ball, and use your hands to lightly pat it out to about 1¼ inches thick. Dip a round biscuit cutter into a little flour and cut out scones from the dough. Put the scones on the baking sheet, spaced a little apart. Brush the tops of the scones with a little milk.

6 Bake for 8–10 minutes until risen and golden. Remove from the oven and place the scones on a wire rack to cool. These freeze really well, so if you want to save some for later in the week, pop a few into some freezer bags.

1⅔ cups self-rising flour, plus extra for kneading

1 teaspoon baking powder

3 tablespoons butter, chilled and cut into small pieces

a handful each of 2 of the following: grated cheese, fresh herbs (finely chopped), sun-dried tomatoes (chopped), olives (pitted and cut in half), ham or bacon (chopped and cooked)

½–⅔ cup milk, plus a little extra for glazing

makes 8 large or 12 small scones

a round biscuit cutter

a baking sheet, greased

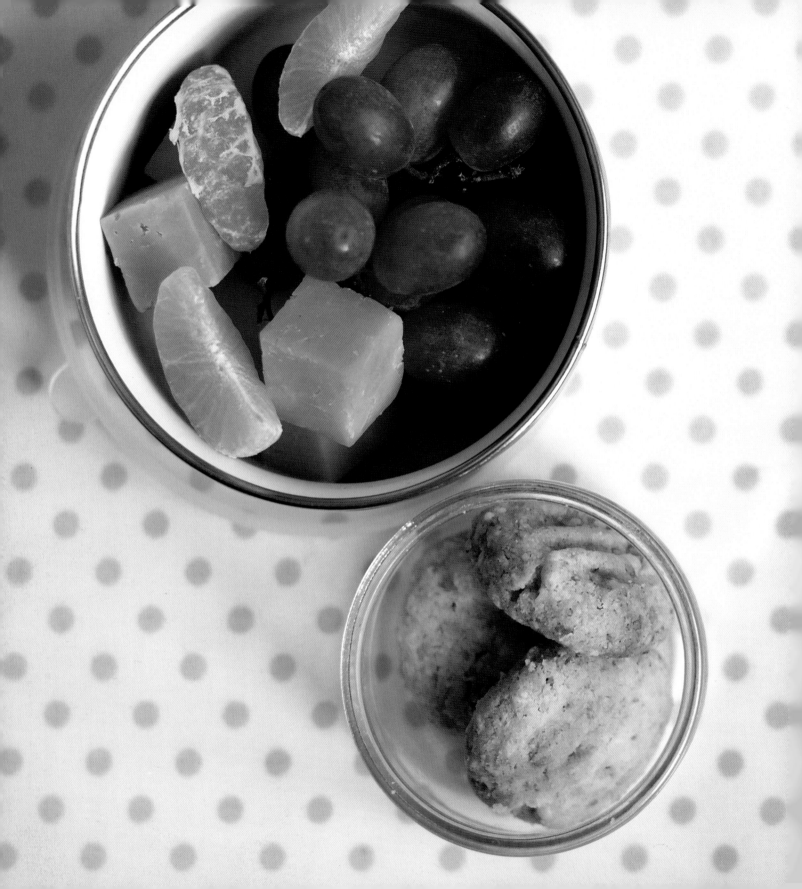

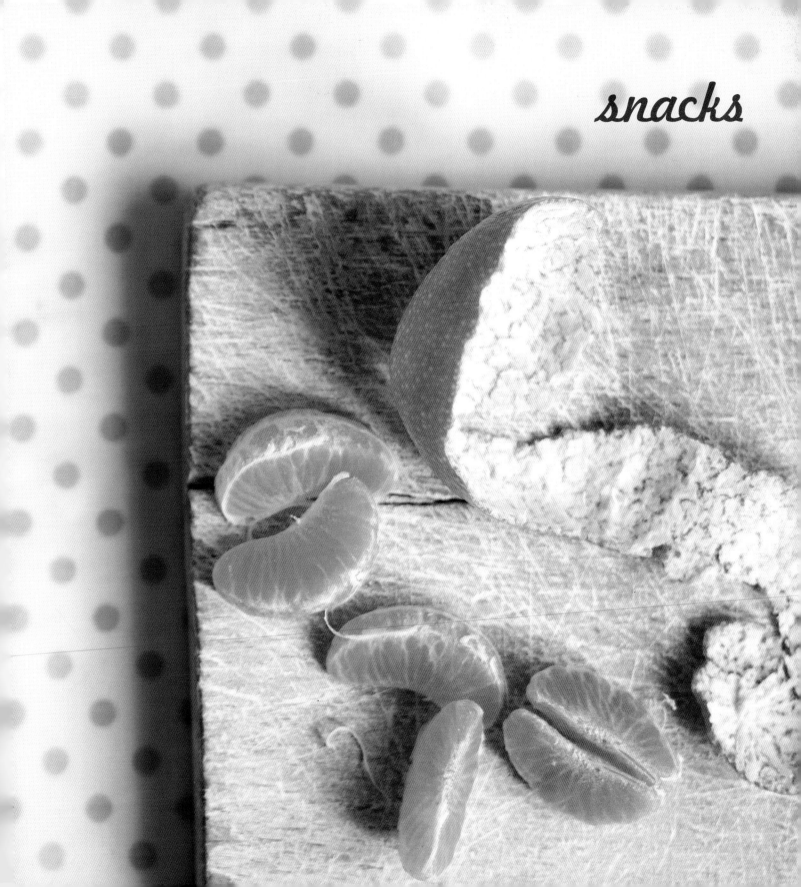

snacks

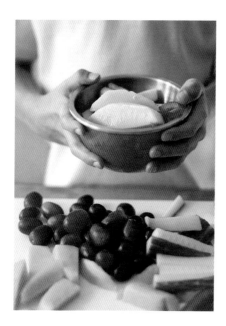

# pack a snack

### which snacks to pack

Most young children need small snacks in between meals to help keep their energy levels up. Regular meals, with snacks in between, can help prevent blood sugar or energy lows. Schools encourage you to provide a snack for your child for the middle of the morning, and many British schools have banned potato chips and chocolate.

Fruits and vegetables are best, but sometimes children need something slightly more substantial, especially if they are active in sports or staying after school for an activity club.

If you are looking in the grocery stores for snacks, be aware that many snacks marketed at children are often heavily refined and high in fat and sugar. These snacks not only lack a variety of important nutrients, but they are also likely to make children feel full, which can put them off eating their next meal.

### keeping it fresh

Children 5 years and over should be eating 5 servings of fresh fruit and vegetables per day to get plenty of vitamins, minerals, fiber, and phytochemicals (plant nutrients)—all of which are essential for a healthy immune system, gut, and heart.

### good fruit

Each fruit contains different nutrients, so work hard to introduce new fruit into your child's diet. Bananas, apples, pears, oranges, plums, grapes, raspberries, strawberries, peaches, and kiwi are all popular fruits for lunchboxes.

Encourage your child to try new fruits by doing the following:
■ Cut kiwis in half and pack a spoon, so they can be eaten like a hard-cooked egg!
■ Cut oranges into quarters, so your child can suck the juice out—boys are often impressed to hear this is a popular snack at half-time among soccer players!

### good vegetables

Good vegetables for snacks include strips of raw bell peppers, cherry tomatoes, and also carrot, celery, or cucumber sticks.

### snack ideas

#### rainbow carton

To help encourage your child to eat a variety of fruits and vegetables, fill an airtight carton with a colorful mix of his/her favorites. Use any fruits and vegetables (preferably seasonal) that you have on hand, and divide the carton up into quarters, putting red grapes, sticks of cucumber, slices of mango, and slices of red bell pepper in each corner.

#### dried fruits

Be creative with your packaging and put raisins, dried apricots, and dried mango into small bags decorated with stickers. Let your child help, so that he/she gets enthusiastic about the contents of his/her lunchbox.

#### medley of mixed dried fruits

There are many dried fruits available, but the combination popular in our house is the medley of dried tropical fruits. Mix together some dried mango, dried pineapple, and papaya in a small airtight carton. For a treat, ask your child to help you half-dip some dried fruit in melted chocolate. Let them dry and give them as a special treat.

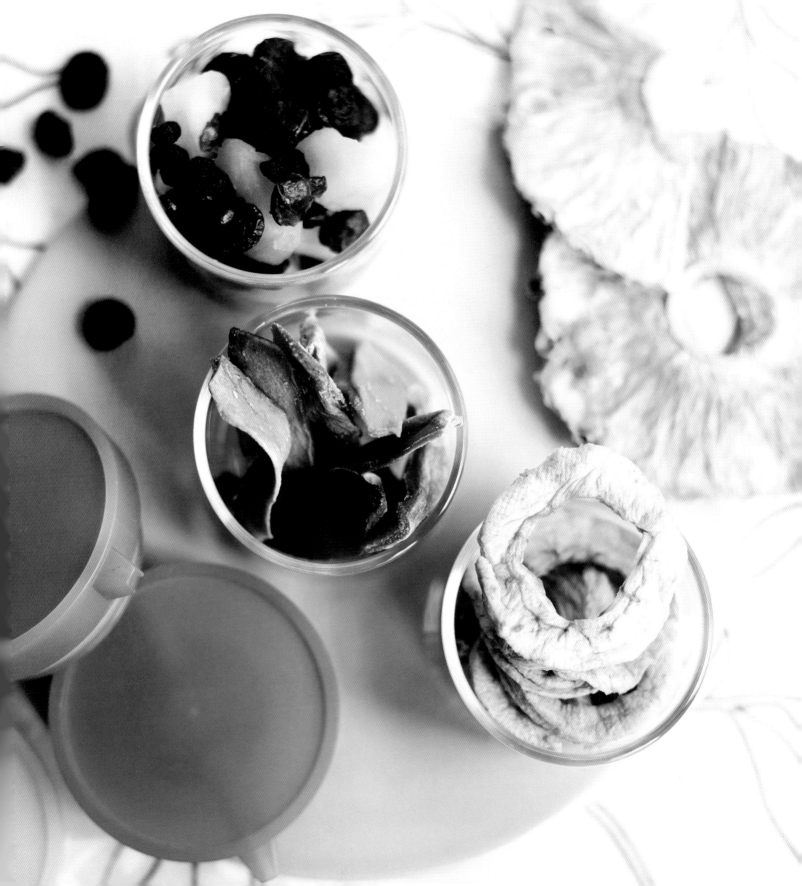

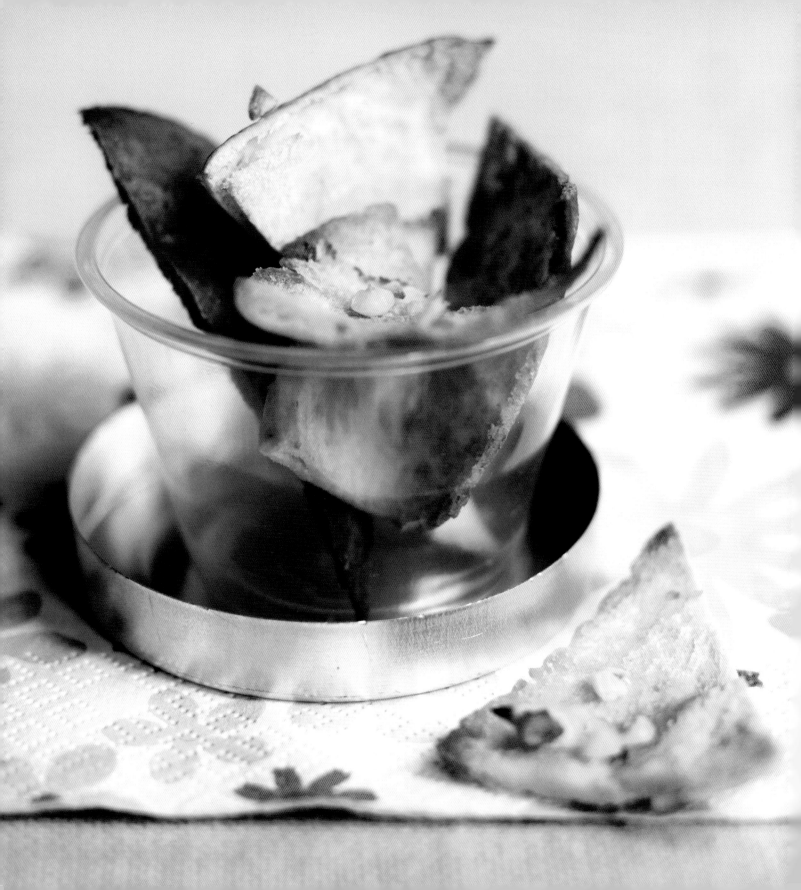

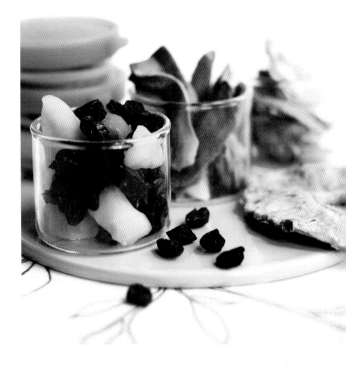

### nuts & seeds

These contain beneficial monounsaturated fats and useful fiber, and are a great healthy snack option. Mix together a handful of dried fruits with some nuts and seeds and pop them in a small carton.

### breadsticks, rice cakes, or cheese biscuits

These are all great, especially with a chunk of cheese and a piece of fresh fruit, and are a good source of carbohydrate.

### garlic pita crisps (see left)

A really simple recipe, children will love biting into these crispy little toasts.

serves 2

2 pita breads

olive oil

garlic clove, crushed

Cut the pita in half lengthwise, cut each half widthwise and then cut each quarter in half diagonally to make 8 triangles. Put the triangles on a baking sheet, drizzle with a little oil, and scatter the garlic on top. Bake for 5–6 minutes until crisp and golden around the edges.

### pieces of cheese

Mini Babybels are often popular with children, partly, I am sure, because of the red waxy coating. Cheese is an excellent source of protein and calcium.

### plain yogurts with toppings

A small carton of yogurt can fill a hungry hole and help keep your child happy until the next meal. If you are buying fruit yogurts, check the label first. I have seen some yogurts for children that contain 2½ teaspoons of sugar in one carton (see page 10 for sugar intake information). For some great topping ideas, see page 102.

### cereal bars

Look at the labels of so-called healthy cereal bars marketed at children—they often contain totally unacceptable levels of fat, salt, and sugar (see pages 10–11 for information on sugar and salt intake). If you can set some time aside, it is much better to make your own cereal bars—see page 120.

**nutrition tip** Garlic is antiviral, antifungal, and antibacterial. Children often love the taste of garlic and these crisps are quicker to eat than garlic bread.

Dips do not have to be complicated, and most children will be happy with a small carton of cream cheese and a handful of breadsticks for dipping. You will need to invest in a little reusable container with a cover, so your child can take the dips to school.

# easy dips

## cream cheese dip

Take 3 heaped tablespoons thick live plain yogurt and mix with 2 tablespoons soft herb and garlic cream cheese (e.g., Boursin). Serve with pita crisps or vegetable sticks.

## chickpea dip

There is very little point in making a small portion of hummus, it is much better to make enough for a few people and keep it in the fridge until needed. You may enjoy eating this for your lunch, too. It is easy to forget about eating good food yourself when you are busy looking after children.

**serves 4**

2 tablespoons sesame seeds

1 teaspoon ground cumin

15-oz. can chickpeas, drained (about 1½–2 cups drained) and rinsed

1 garlic clove, finely chopped

freshly squeezed juice of 1 lemon

3 tablespoons olive oil

a handful of fresh cilantro, chopped

freshly ground black pepper

a few sticks of vegetables (e.g., carrots, cucumber, and celery)

Heat the sesame seeds and ground cumin in a dry skillet for a minute to release their flavor, and put into a bowl (or food processor). Add the chickpeas, garlic, lemon juice, and oil and whiz or mash until pureed.

Add the cilantro and freshly ground black pepper and stir in or whiz again. If necessary, add a little more olive oil or water until it's the consistency you want.

Serve a small bowl of hummus with some vegetable sticks for dipping.

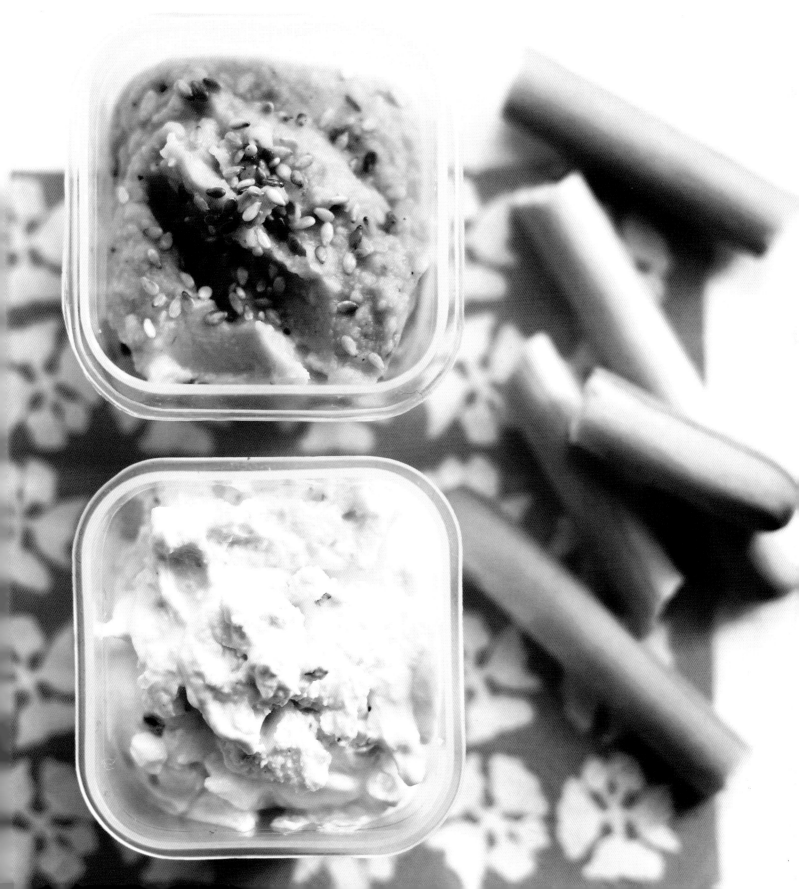

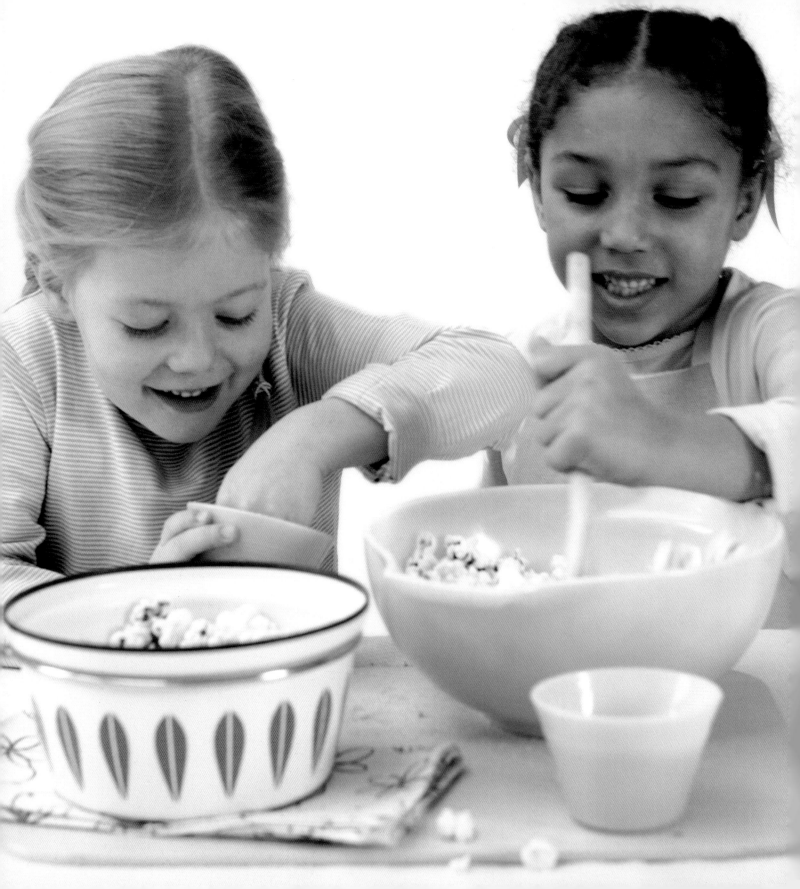

Store-bought popcorn can contain very high amounts of sugar or salt. It is cheaper and healthier to make your own. Children are fascinated by the change in size and shape of corn kernels before and after they have popped—make sure you show them. Let them listen to the sound of the popping corn in the saucepan.

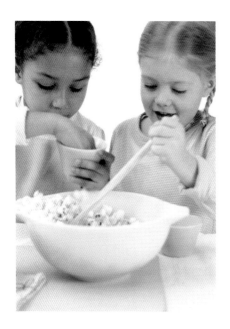

# butter popcorn

**1** Put the oil into a large lightweight pot with a fitted lid and heat until it is hot.

**2** Tip the kernels into the pot, and shake the pot gently over the heat to coat the kernels.

**3** When the kernels start to pop, continue shaking the pot until the popping subsides—this will take a few minutes.

**4** Remove from the heat, uncover, and pour the butter (if using) over it. Sprinkle with salt (or sugar). Stir gently with a wooden spoon and tip into a serving bowl.

**Other good things you could try with popcorn:** Vanilla sugar instead of ordinary sugar, or light brown sugar for a more toffee-like flavor, 1 tablespoon of maple syrup, or mix a pinch of cinnamon into your sugar. For savory popcorn, try adding ½ cup finely grated cheddar or Parmesan.

2 tablespoons sunflower oil

⅓ cup popcorn kernels

2 tablespoons butter, melted (optional)

salt, to taste (or a sprinkling of sugar for a sweet treat)

**serves** 2

**nutrition tip** This is an ideal snack food as long as you **don't** add lots of sugar! Popcorn contains fiber and is low in fat, and is a much healthier snack alternative to chips.

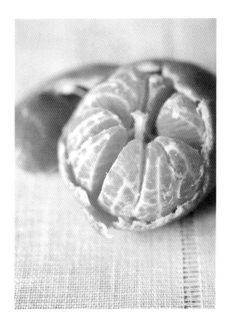

You can either give these as an alternative to sandwiches with some crunchy vegetable sticks, as a snack, or serve with a piece of cheese and some fruit.

# cheese & seed savory cookies

1 cup grated cheddar

½ cup (1 stick) minus 1 tablespoon butter, softened

1 scant cup all-purpose flour

1 teaspoon baking powder

1 tablespoon sunflower seeds

1 cup puffed rice (breakfast cereal)

*2 baking sheets*

**makes** about 20

**nutrition tip** Cheese provides calcium, which is needed for building healthy bones. It is a good snack and the ideal alternative to a sweet dessert.

**1** Preheat the oven to 350°F.

**2** Line the baking sheets with baking parchment.

**3** Put the cheese and butter in a mixing bowl. Add the flour, baking powder, and seeds.

**4** Put the puffed rice (breakfast cereal) into a plastic bag and use a rolling pin to roll over the bag and break up the rice. Add to the bowl and mix everything together. This will take some time and you will need to use your hands.

**5** Squeeze the mixture into small balls, about the size of cherry tomatoes. Place on the baking sheets and flatten slightly with a fork.

**6** Bake for 10–15 minutes, until light golden. Carefully transfer the savory cookies to a wire rack to cool.

**7** Let cool completely, then store in an airtight container or freeze.

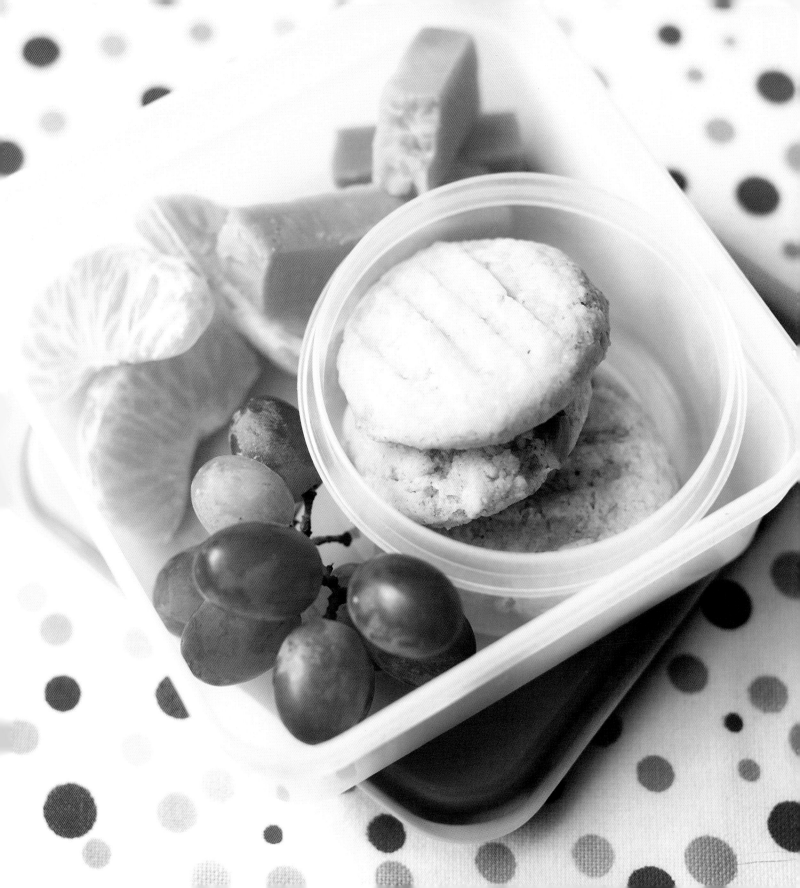

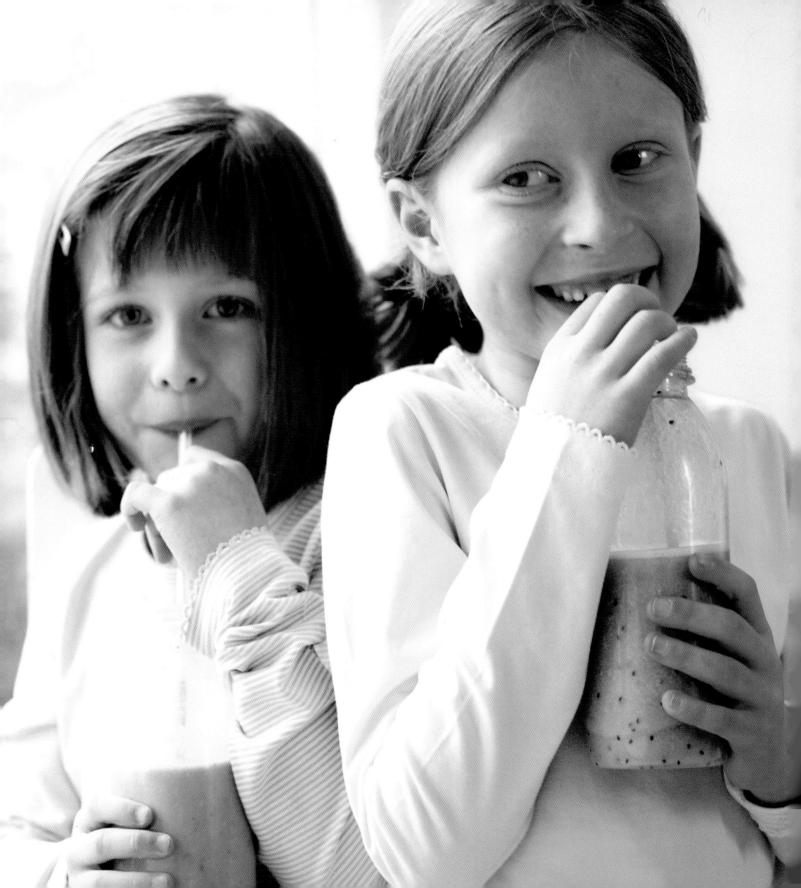

# smoothie trio

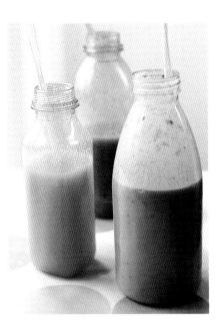

I make these smoothies most mornings—they only take a couple of minutes. Just chop up any fruit that you have to hand, add some juice and blend. Use old fruit juice bottles and pack with a colorful straw. Use these basic recipes to start.

## tropical mix

Pour 2 big glasses of orange or pineapple juice into a blender or food processor. Slice a mango either side of the flat pit, peel, then roughly cut the flesh, and add to the juice. Add a few pieces of canned or fresh pineapple or 1 passion fruit and blend until smooth.

## pink milk

This will need to be kept cold—invest in a good thermos.

Pour 2 big glasses of milk into a blender. Add 1 ripe banana, 2 big handfuls of raspberries or strawberries, and a little honey, then blend until smooth.

## green juice

Pour 2 big glasses of apple juice into a blender or food processor. Peel a ripe kiwi and cut the flesh into pieces, then add to the juice along with 1 peeled and roughly chopped banana. Blend until smooth. Chill all smoothies before serving.

**nutrition tip** Smoothies are easier to make than you might think and are a great way of encouraging your children to eat fruit, and even vegetables, as well as increase their fluid intake. They contain a large amount of natural sugar, so are great served alongside cereal or toast.

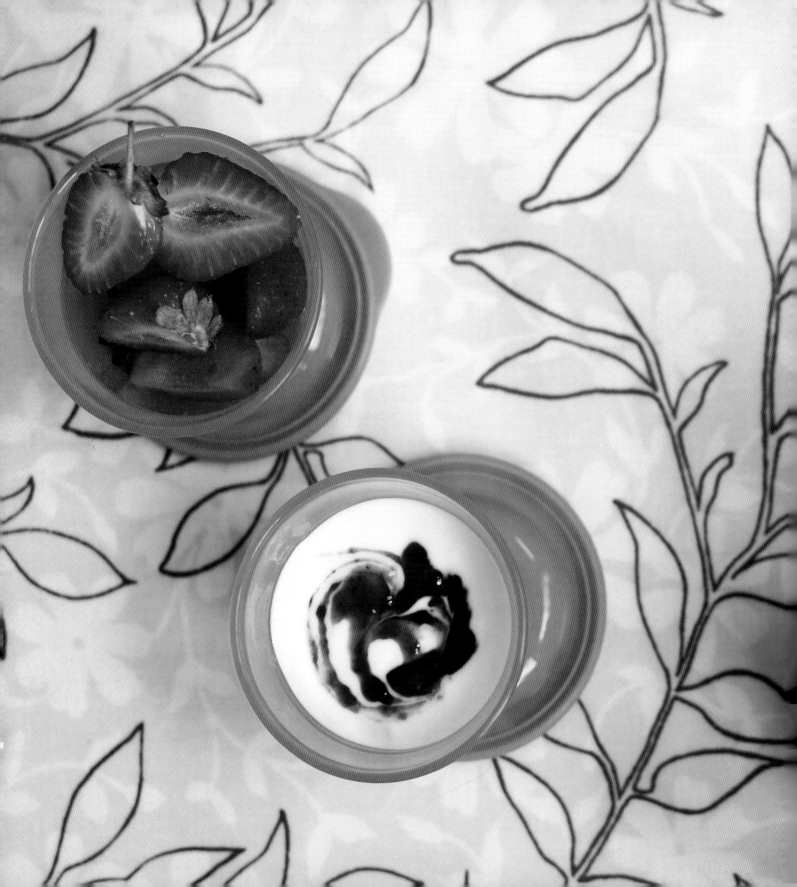

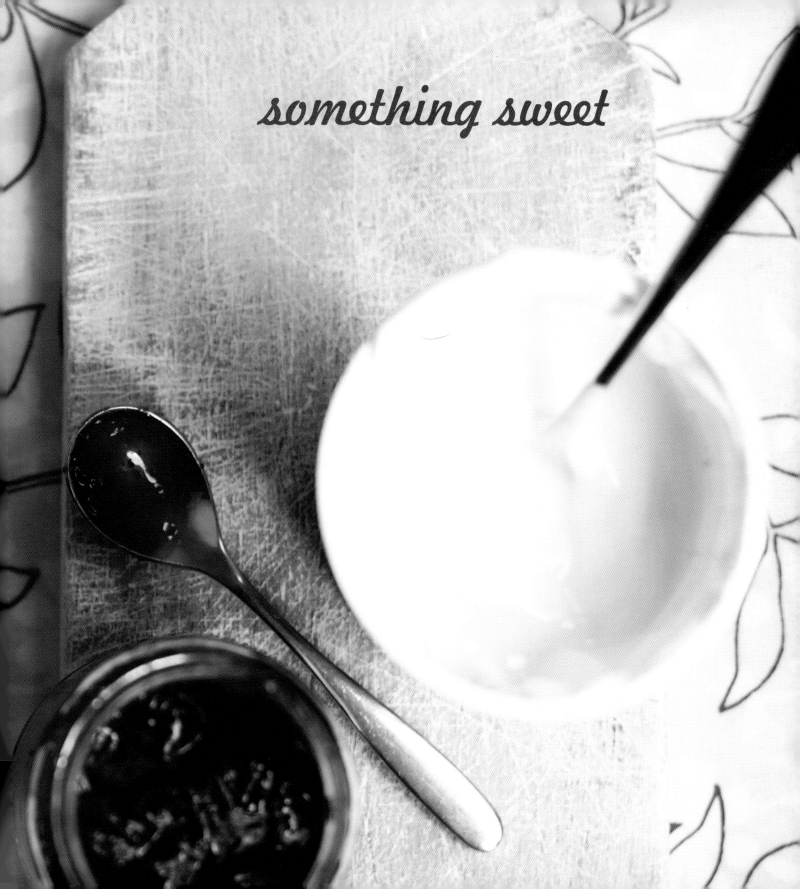

something sweet

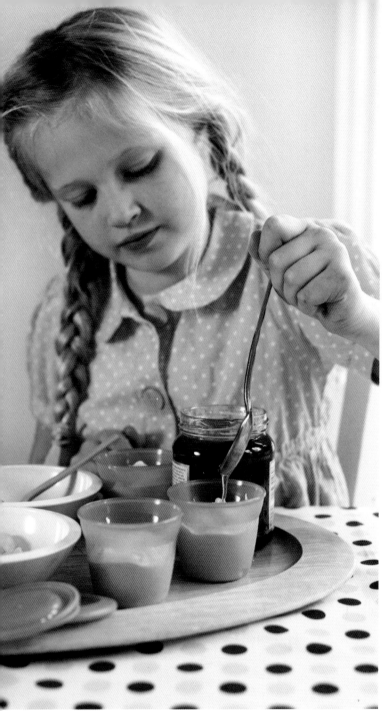

# yogurt pots

You may, like me, be fed up with the high amount of sugar, additives, and preservatives that can be found in so many of the yogurts aimed at children.

I believe the best answer is to invest in some little plastic cartons with tight-fitting lids and create your own yogurts. It takes no time at all to spoon some plain yogurt and a spoonful of jam or honey into a container. Just don't forget to pack a spoon too. Adding your own flavorings to plain yogurt can also work out to be much less expensive.

Plain probiotic yogurt is best, because it contains friendly bacteria that are good for your child's gut. It is believed that the friendly bacteria can help to prevent constipation and diarrhea as well as food poisoning.

It is also a good idea to use whole-milk yogurt. Children do need some fat in their diet, and whole-milk plain yogurt actually only contains 3 g fat per 100 g.

The following pages contain some ideas to get you started. Fill your small carton three quarters full with plain probiotic yogurt and top with one of the ideas listed to the right. When you add a topping to your plain yogurt, try not to add too much or you could end up going over your child's daily sugar allowance (see page 11). Children don't need sugar, and should get used to the natural sweetness of dried fruit.

### apricots & honey

Finely chop 3 dried apricots, and add to plain yogurt along with 1 teaspoon honey.

### jam with fresh fruit

Add 1 teaspoon fresh fruit jam to plain yogurt along with a handful of fresh or frozen raspberries or other berries.

### apple & raisins

Core and peel an eating apple, then grate it and mix with a tiny bit of lemon juice to stop it from going brown. Add to plain yogurt along with a handful of raisins or dried cranberries.

### banana

Mash or finely chop 1 very ripe banana. You might like to mix it with a tiny bit of lemon juice to stop it from going brown. Add it to plain yogurt. If your child likes dates, add a few of these, chopped.

### apple puree

Core and peel 4 dessert apples, chop, and put into a saucepan with a tiny dribble of water. Cook gently until the apples are soft. Taste, and if they are really tart add a little light brown sugar. Add to the yogurt. This will make enough for 3 or 4 portions.

### muesli with honey

Sprinkle a handful of muesli on top of plain yogurt and drizzle with a little honey.

If you are going to make a cake, you may as well make a big one. At least that way it will last for a few packed lunches. People always comment on how moist this cake is. My secret is to add orange juice to the raisins to make them plump and juicy.

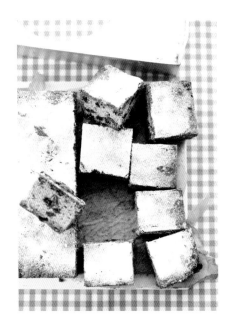

# golden raisin cake

1. Preheat the oven to 325°F.

2. Put the raisins in a saucepan and cover with the orange juice. Bring to a boil, reduce the heat slightly, and cook for 15 minutes or until all the juice has been absorbed by the raisins.

3. Add the butter to the raisins and stir gently over low heat until the butter has melted. Remove from the heat.

4. Mix the eggs, sugar, and vanilla extract in a large mixing bowl.

5. Add the raisins, flour, and baking powder to the egg mixture and mix thoroughly. Pour into the roasting pan.

6. Bake for about 1 hour. You will need to check the cake after 40–45 minutes, when you may like to cover the top with foil to stop it from going too brown.

7. Leave the cake in the pan for 5 minutes and then cut into about 24 squares. Dust with confectioners' sugar.

1 lb (about 3¼ cups) golden raisins

about 1 cup orange juice

1 cup plus 2 tablespoons (2¼ sticks) butter

3 eggs

1¼ cups light brown sugar

2 teaspoons vanilla extract

2¾ cups self-rising flour

1 teaspoon baking powder

confectioners' sugar, to dust (optional)

**makes** about 24 squares

*a 12 x 8-inch roasting pan, greased and lined with baking parchment (or dusted with flour)*

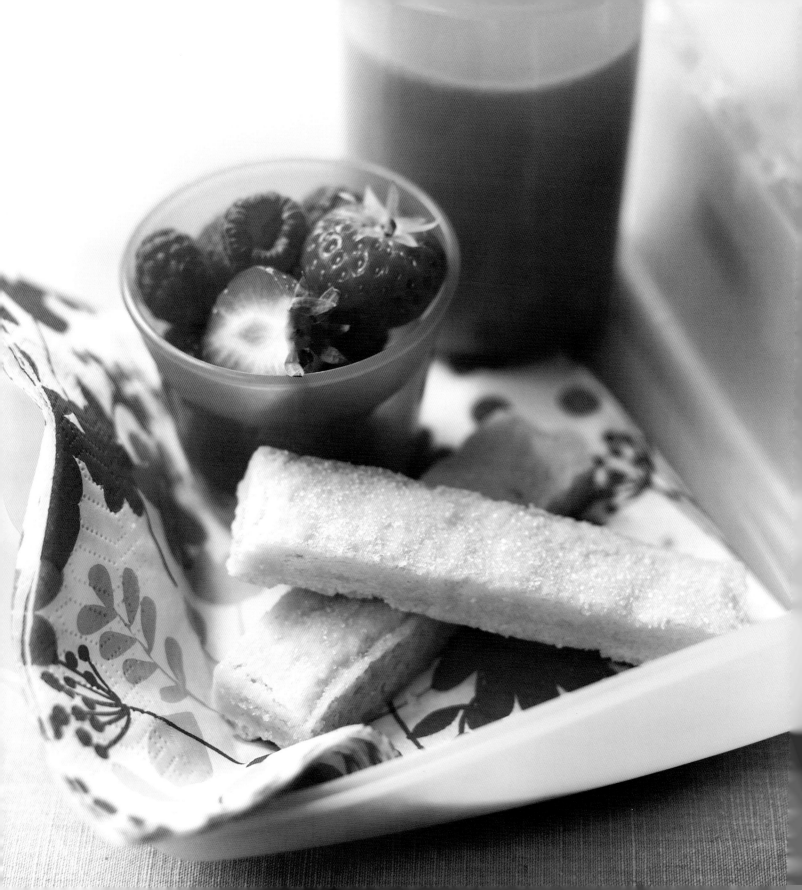

A slice of homemade shortbread with some fresh berries is an ideal dessert for a summer lunchbox. If your children are keen on lemon, then add the zest of 2 lemons instead of just the 1, for a real zing. Or if they prefer orange, try adding the zest from 1 orange instead.

# lemon shortbread with berries

1. Preheat the oven to 375°F.

2. Beat the butter and sugar together until soft, pale, and fluffy.

3. Add the lemon zest, flour, and cornstarch and mix again until it comes together.

4. Cover the bowl and chill the mixture for 10 minutes, if you have the time. If not, you can bake it right away—it will not make a big difference either way.

5. Press the dough into the prepared pan and bake for 15 minutes.

6. Remove from the oven and dust with sugar, if liked. Score the dough into about 12 sticks (score in half and then score each half into about 6 sticks) and let cool completely in the pan.

7. Once cooled, cut out the slices and remove from the pan. Store in an airtight container.

¾ cup (1½ sticks) butter, softened

⅓ cup sugar, plus extra to dust

zest of 1 unwaxed lemon

1½ cups all-purpose flour

½ cup cornstarch

fresh seasonal fruit, for serving

**makes** 10–12 shortbread sticks

*an 8-inch-square pan, greased and lined with baking parchment (or dusted with flour)*

**nutrition tip** Whenever you give your child something sweet, like cookies, cakes, or shortbread, try to always offer some fresh fruit alongside to help boost their vitamin and mineral intake.

# cranberry cookies

You can make your own variations of these by adding other chopped dried fruits or chocolate. They will stay fresh in an airtight container for a week and they also freeze really well. These cookies should be crisp and firm like shortbread, not gooey.

½ cup (1 stick) minus 1 tablespoon butter, softened

½ cup sugar

1 egg, beaten

½ teaspoon vanilla extract

2 cups all-purpose flour

a good ⅓ cup dried cranberries, raisins, chopped apricots, or finely chopped milk chocolate

**makes** 30–32

*a large cookie sheet, greased*

1. Preheat the oven to 350°F.

2. Beat together the butter and sugar until pale and fluffy. Beat in the egg, then add the vanilla extract.

3. Add the flour and cranberries and mix together. Use your hands to mold the mixture into a big ball.

4. Break the dough into three equal balls and roll each one into a log, about 4 inches in diameter. Slice each log into about 10 cookies. Place on the cookie sheet and bake for 9–11 minutes or until just golden around the edges.

# chocolate chip cookies

Get your children involved with this recipe—they will love mixing everything together and then spooning the mixture onto the baking sheets. These are a great alternative to a bar of chocolate.

⅓ cup (about ¾ stick) butter, softened

⅓ cup light brown sugar

a few drops of vanilla extract

1 egg

2 tablespoons corn syrup

1 cup plus 2 tablespoons self-rising flour

2½ oz. chocolate, cut into small pieces or a scant ½ cup chocolate chips

**makes** 20

*a large cookie sheet, greased*

1. Preheat the oven to 350°F.

2. Cream the butter and sugar together until really soft. Add the vanilla extract and egg and beat again. Add the syrup and mix together.

3. Add the flour and mix together, then add the chocolate chunks and mix well.

4. Take small spoonfuls of the mixture and mold into balls about the size of walnuts.

5. Place on the cookie sheet, flatten their tops slightly with a knife or fork, and bake for about 6 minutes. Remove from the oven and let cool. The cookies will continue to set as they cool.

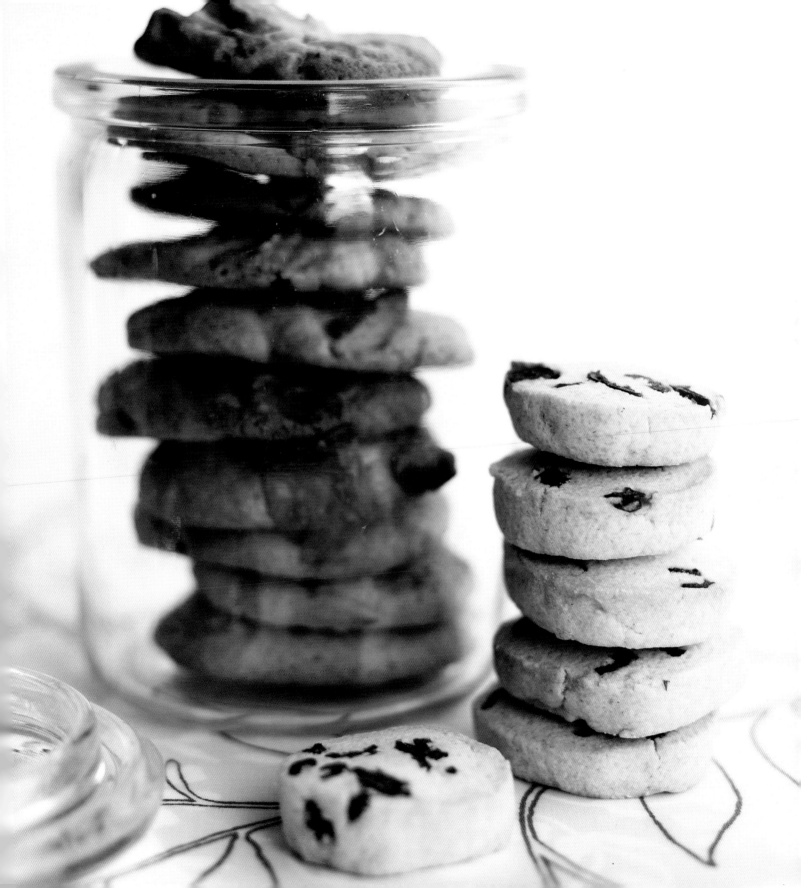

# muffins

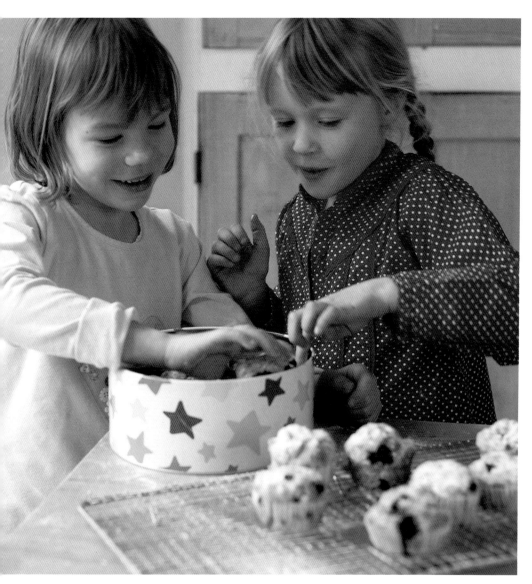

I developed this recipe to make 12 muffins, so if you only need 6 you can freeze the other half to use another week. It's nice to send your child to school with homemade baked treats, especially if it's a recipe that's been in the family for generations, like this one. Experiment with different fruit —a little pureed pear or apple or mashed banana can be just as delicious as a handful of berries.

3½ tablespoons butter (or sunflower oil)

2⅓ cups self-rising flour

2 teaspoons baking powder

a heaping ⅓ cup sugar

2 eggs

½ cup plain yogurt (if you don't have yogurt, you could use milk)

½ cup milk

a few drops of vanilla extract

2 big handfuls of berries (e.g., blueberries or raspberries)

**makes 12**

*a 12-holed muffin pan*

*12 paper muffin cups*

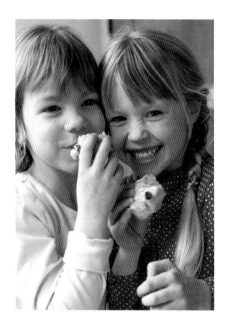

# william's mini tarts

The classic sweet pastry I use in this recipe is light, crisp, and easy to make. I use it for most of my sweet tarts and pies. My daughter's friend William came up with the idea of adding thinly sliced apple and golden syrup to the tart cases when he was making jam tarts one day. They really are delicious.

**for the pastry:**

1¾ cups all-purpose flour, plus extra for dusting

½ cup (1 stick) butter, chilled and cut into small pieces

1 teaspoon sugar

1 egg yolk

1–2 tablespoons cold water

*a round pastry cutter*

*an 18-holed tart pan, greased*

**makes 18**

**for the fillings:**

**for each mini apple tart:**

a few thin slices of dessert apple

1–2 teaspoons corn syrup

**for each mini lemon tart:**

1–2 teaspoons lemon curd

**for each mini jam tart:**

1–2 teaspoons jam of your choice

1. Preheat the oven 400°F. Line the 12 muffin holes with muffin cups—if you don't have any, just grease the muffin holes really well with butter.

2. Melt the butter in the microwave or in a small pan. Let cool slightly and set aside. Sift the flour and baking powder in a large bowl. Add the sugar to the flour.

3. In a small bowl, whisk the eggs with a fork, then add the yogurt, milk, vanilla extract, and melted butter.

4. Quickly and gently mix everything together in the large bowl. Don't overmix or your muffins will not be light. Quickly fold in the fruit, and then spoon the mixture into the muffin cups.

5. Bake for 25–30 minutes or until well risen and golden brown. Take the muffins out of the pan and leave to cool on a wire rack. When they have completely cooled, place in an airtight container, or you could bag, label, and freeze half for another time.

1. Sift the flour into a large mixing bowl, add the butter, and rub it in using your fingertips until the mixture looks like fine bread crumbs. Stir in the sugar. Use the knife to mix in the egg yolk, then add the water, a little at a time, stirring with the knife until the mixture comes together and you can form a ball with your hands.

2. Wrap the dough in plastic wrap and put it in the fridge for 30 minutes—this will make it easier to roll out.

3. Preheat the oven to 400°F. Sprinkle both the counter and your rolling pin with a little flour and roll the dough out to about ⅛-inch thick. Dip the cutter in flour, then cut out as many circles as you can—gather the remaining dough scraps; you want 18 circles in all. Lay the pie shells in the tart pan and press them gently into place. Prick the bottom of each crust once with a fork.

4. Put the tart pan into the oven. Bake for 6 minutes until the crusts are very pale golden. Remove from the oven. For the apple tarts, carefully put a few slices of dessert apple into each pie shell and drizzle with the syrup. Alternatively, add the filling of your choice and put the pan back into the oven for 6 minutes.

5. Remove from the oven. Let the tarts cool for a few minutes, then use a butter knife to gently lift them out of the pan. Let them cool completely on a wire rack.

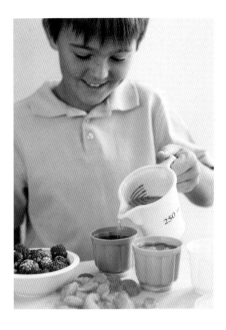

Jello is something all children enjoy, so why not put some in their lunchbox as a tangy treat? Add some seasonal fresh fruits or canned fruits into the cups before you pour over the jello. You can also make the jello with a combination of fruit juice and water.

# fresh fruit jellos

**orange jello:**

1 package orange jello

1 can oranges or fresh tangerines

**raspberry jello:**

1 package raspberry jello

1 can raspberries or fresh or frozen raspberries

**lemon jello:**

1 package lemon jello

1 can citrus fruits or fresh orange, peach, or apricots

**strawberry jello:**

1 package strawberry jello

fresh or frozen strawberries or raspberries

*5–6 jello molds*

**makes** each package of jello make 2 cups (16 fl. oz.)

**1** Prepare the jello according to the package instructions. If you are using canned fruits, prepare the jello as normal, but substitute the fruit-flavored liquid from the can for some of the water called for in the jello recipe.

**2** Mash half the canned or fresh fruit to a pulp and add to the jello mixture. Divide the remaining fruits between the jello molds. Pour the jello and mashed fruit mixture over the fruit in each mold and let set overnight or until firm.

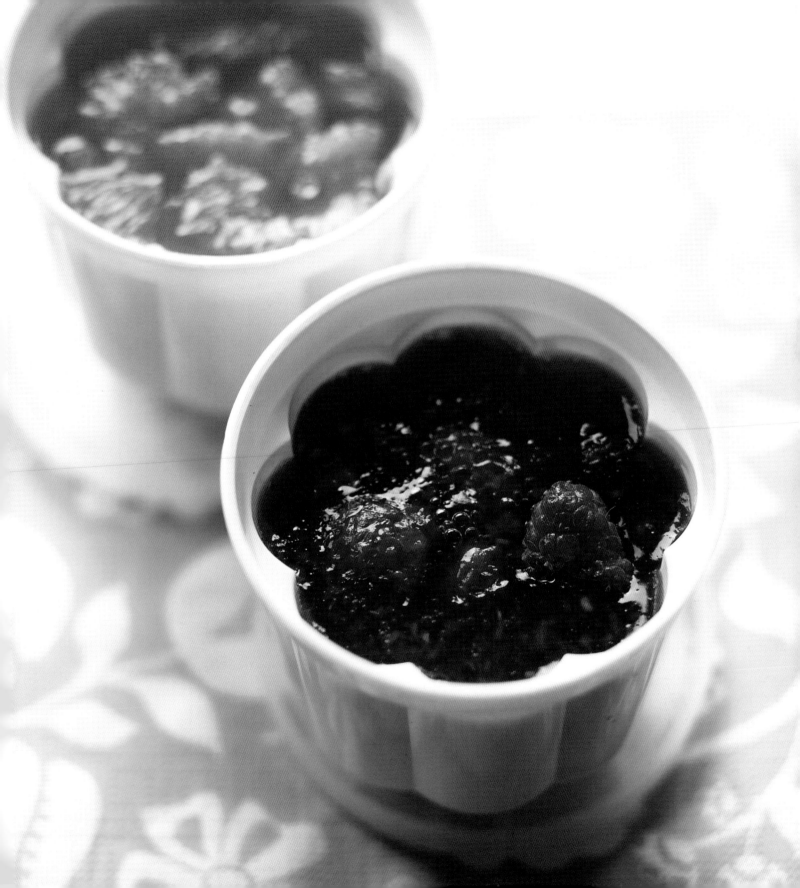

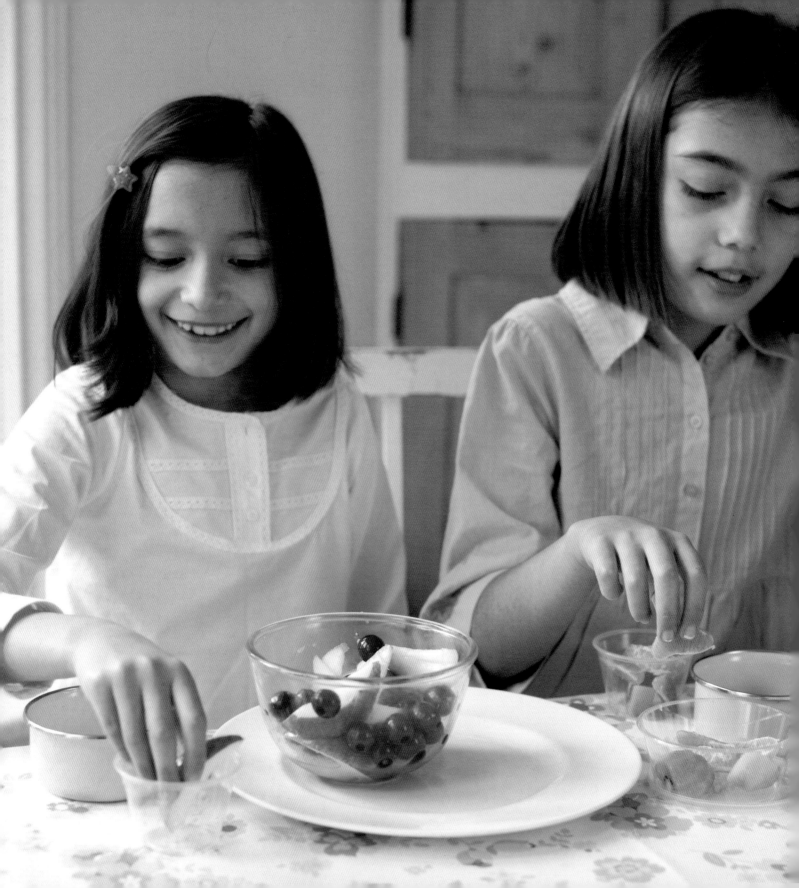

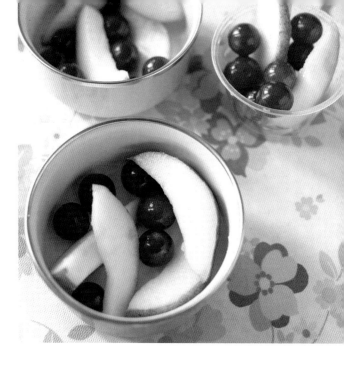

Sometimes all you need to do is change the packaging of food to entice children to start eating it. Some children find a variety of fresh fruit, chopped and mixed together in a cup, more appealing than eating whole individual fruits. Mixing familiar fruit with something new can be a great way to introduce different fruit to your child's diet.

# little cups of fresh fruits

★ **kiwi & satsuma**

Peel the skin off a kiwi using a sharp knife and cut the flesh into bite-size chunks. Peel a satsuma or tangerine and mix the segments with the kiwi chunks in an airtight container.

★ **pineapple & mango**

Tropical fruits are often popular with children. Cut them into big pieces that they can hold, or small pieces that they can eat with a fork. Peel and cut a pineapple into bite-size chunks. Put a handful in an airtight container and store the rest in the fridge for later. Peel and cut half a mango into bite-size chunks. Put a handful into the airtight container of pineapple and mix together. Store the other half in the fridge for later.

★ **grapes & pear**

Core a pear and cut into bite-size chunks, then sprinkle with a little freshly squeezed lemon juice to prevent it from turning brown. Put the pears into a container and add a handful of grapes.

**nutrition tip** Sometimes it is easier to eat fruit that is chopped up and ready to eat, but try to vary this with whole fruit so that children become used to eating fruit right from the tree. Children should be eating 5 a day!

As a busy mom, I often bake 2 cakes at the same time and pop one in the freezer to eat a week later. It takes exactly the same amount of time to make 2 of these gingerbread cakes as it does to make 1. Alternatively, this cake mix can be baked in one 25-cm-round cake pan, but it will need to cook for 1½ hours.

1 cup (2 sticks) butter

1 cup dark brown sugar

⅔ cup black treacle or molasses

2 eggs, beaten

12 oz. (about 2½–2⅔ cups) all-purpose flour

2 teaspoons ground cinnamon

1 tablespoon ground ginger

1 teaspoon baking soda

1¼ cups warm milk

**makes** 2 x 2 lb loaves

*2 x 2-lb loaf pans, greased and lined with baking parchment*

# sticky gingerbread

1   Preheat the oven to 275˚F.

2   Line the 2 loaf pans with baking parchment.

3   Put the butter, sugar, and treacle into a large saucepan and heat gently, stirring constantly until melted.

4   Remove from the heat, let cool slightly, and then stir in the beaten eggs.

5   Sift the flour, cinnamon, and ginger into the melted mixture.

6   Mix together the baking soda and warm milk. Add to the ginger mixture, mix well, and pour equal amounts of the mixture into each pan.

7   Bake for just under 1 hour. The top of the cake will be slightly golden with a lovely crust and a skewer should come out clean.

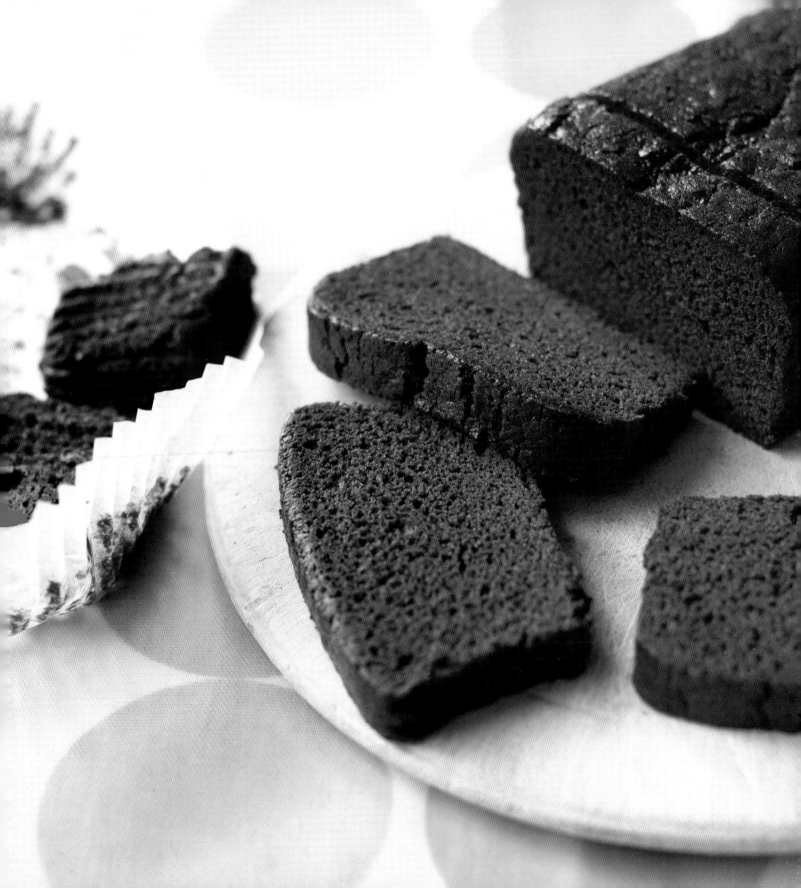

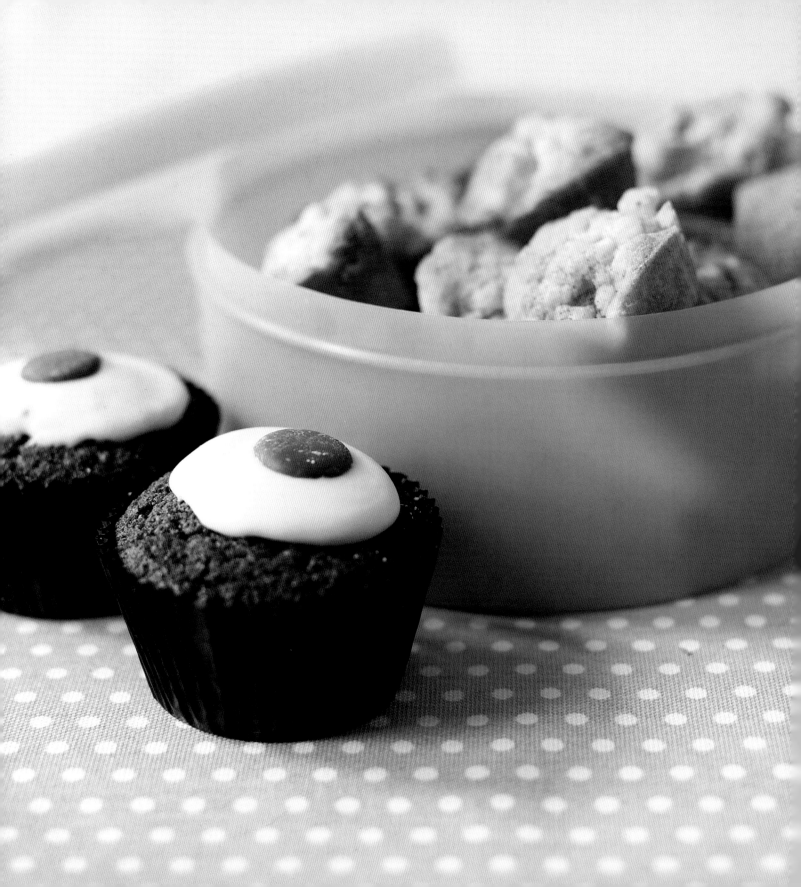

# chocolate cupcakes

These are ideal for a Friday treat. There are many ways to decorate mini cupcakes—let your children decide how.

¾ cup (1½ sticks) unsalted butter, softened

¾ cup sugar

3 large eggs, beaten

1⅓ cups (minus 2 tablespoons) self-rising flour

2 tablespoons cocoa powder

about 2 tablespoons milk

1⅔ cups confectioners' sugar

pink food coloring

chocolate buttons, for decorating

*2 x 12-holed mini muffin pans*

*24 paper cups*

**makes** 24 mini cupcakes

1. Preheat the oven to 350°F.

2. Put the paper cups into the holes of the mini muffin pans. Cream together the butter and sugar until pale and fluffy. Gradually add the eggs, one at a time, beating well after each addition.

3. Fold the flour and cocoa powder into the mixture. Then add enough milk, so that the batter drops easily from the spoon. Fill the paper cups with spoonfuls of the mixture. Bake for 10 minutes. Remove from the oven, take the cupcakes out of the pan, and let cool on a wire rack.

4. Sift the confectioners' sugar into a bowl and mix with a little hot water until it reaches a thick pouring consistency. Add the pink food coloring and mix.

5. Spread a little icing over the cupcakes and decorate with chocolate buttons. Let them set. Store in an airtight container.

# mini pear cakes

These cakes are very quick to make and freeze excellently. Make sure the pears are nice and ripe before making this recipe.

1 ripe pear or 1 eating apple

½ cup vegetable oil

1 egg

⅓ cup sugar, plus extra for dusting

1 cup all-purpose flour (or ½ cup all-purpose flour and ½ cup wholewheat flour)

1½ teaspoons baking powder

a pinch of salt

ground cinnamon, for dusting

*2 x 12-holed mini muffin pans, greased*

**makes** 24 mini pear cakes

1. Peel the pear, slice it in half, core it and then cut into small pieces.

2. Put the oil, egg, and sugar in a bowl and whisk them together.

3. Add the flour and the pear and quickly mix everything together.

4. Fill each muffin hole two thirds full with the mixture and then bake for 12–15 minutes until risen and light golden.

5. Remove from the oven, take the pear cakes out of the pan, and dust with the cinnamon and let cool on a wire rack.

# muesli cookies

Muesli is a good mix of carbohydrates (oats), protein (nuts), and vitamins (dried fruit), and tastes great in these sweet cookies.

¾ cup (1½ sticks) butter

3 tablespoons honey

2 cups muesli

1½ cups self-rising flour

¼ cup light brown sugar

*2 large cookie sheets, greased*

**makes** about 20

1. Preheat the oven to 350°F.

2. Melt the butter and honey in a saucepan, then remove from the heat.

3. Put the muesli, flour, and sugar into a large bowl and then add the butter mixture. Mix well.

4. Drop spoonfuls of the mixture, spaced apart, onto the lined cookie sheets. Bake for 10–15 minutes or until golden.

5. Remove from the oven, lift them off the cookie sheets, and let cool on a wire rack.

# fruity oat bars

I only make large batches of oat bars because they are very popular in my family. If they don't all disappear after baking, store half in the freezer for lunchbox snacks.

scant ½ cup light brown sugar

¾ cup (1½ sticks) butter

½ cup corn syrup

3 cups rolled oats

½ cup dried apricots, finely chopped (try to buy unsulfered ones if you can)

*a 12 x 8-inch roasting pan, greased and lined with baking parchment*

**makes** 12

1. Preheat the oven to 350°F.

2. Put the sugar, butter, and golden syrup into a pan. Heat gently over low heat until the sugar has dissolved.

3. Remove the pan from the heat, add the oats and apricots, and mix well.

4. Tip the mixture into the prepared pan and spread it out evenly right to the edges. Use the back of the spoon to smooth the top. Bake for 18–20 minutes, until golden and cooked.

5. Remove from the oven and let the oat bars cool for 5 minutes.

6. While the oat bars are still warm, use a knife to mark them into squares. Let them cool completely on a wire rack. Cut them into squares along the score marks and store them in an airtight container.

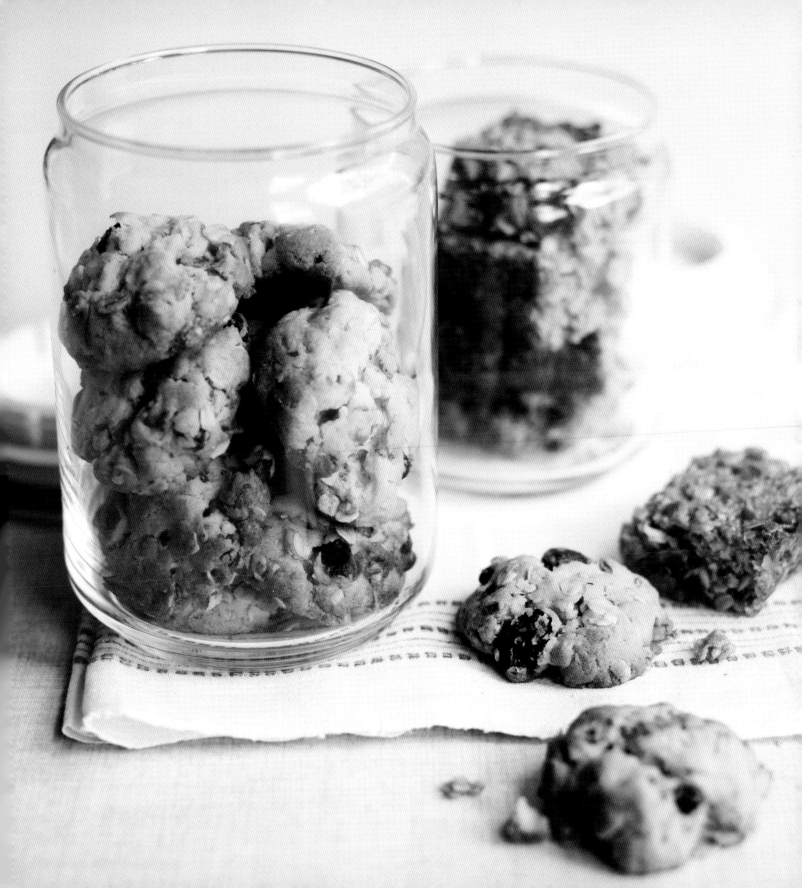

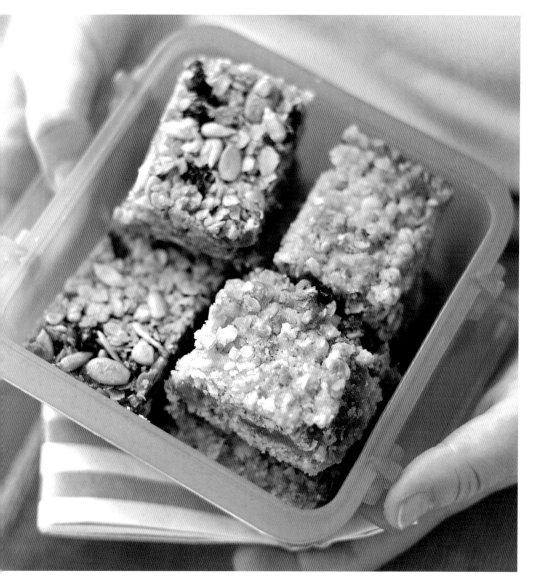

# cereal bars

⅓ cup plus 1½ tablespoons sunflower oil

2½ tablespoons light brown sugar

½ cup corn syrup

2½ cups rolled oats

¾ cup mixture of seeds (e.g. sunflower seeds, pumpkin seeds)

½ cup dried fruits (e.g., raisins, dried cranberries, or chopped apricots)

**makes 16**

*an 8-inch-square pan, greased*

1. Preheat the oven to 350°F.

2. Put the oil, sugar, and syrup into a pan and heat very gently to dissolve the sugar.

3. Add the rest of the ingredients and mix well. Tip into the greased pan and bake for 15–18 minutes until set and golden.

4. Let cool for 10 minutes, and then score into 16 bars.

5. Let cool completely in the pan, then lift out the entire slab, and cut along the score-marks into 16 bars.

6. Store in an airtight container.

**nutrition tip** Oats are a great source of fiber and give long-lasting energy. The seeds are a fantastic source of protein, and the dried fruit contains essential vitamins.

Dried fruit is a great source of fiber and I strongly recommend having a stash of them in your cupboard.

# apricot slices

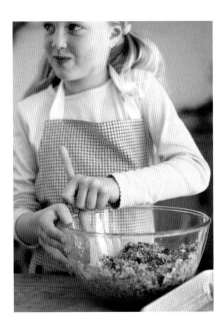

**1** Preheat the oven to 350°F.

**2** Put the dried apricots and orange juice into a small saucepan. Simmer gently for about 15 minutes, until all the juice has been absorbed by the apricots (they should be soft and sticky).

**3** Put the oil and honey into another saucepan and heat gently until the honey dissolves into the oil. Add the oats and flour to the oil and mix.

**4** Put half of the oat mixture into the square pan and press down. Cover with apricots—make sure that you cover the oats with the apricots. Spread the remaining oat mixture over the top of the apricots to cover.

**5** Bake for 20–25 minutes until golden on the top. Remove from the oven and score into 16 slices while still warm. Once cooled, cut the slices along the score lines and store in an airtight container.

1⅓ cups dried apricots (try to buy unsulfered ones if you can), finely chopped

about 6 tablespoons orange juice —you may need to add a little more during cooking

¾ cup sunflower oil

¼ cup honey

1¾ cups oats

1⅓ cups all-purpose flour (or a mixture of wholemeal and plain flour)

*an 8-inch-square pan, greased*

**makes 16**

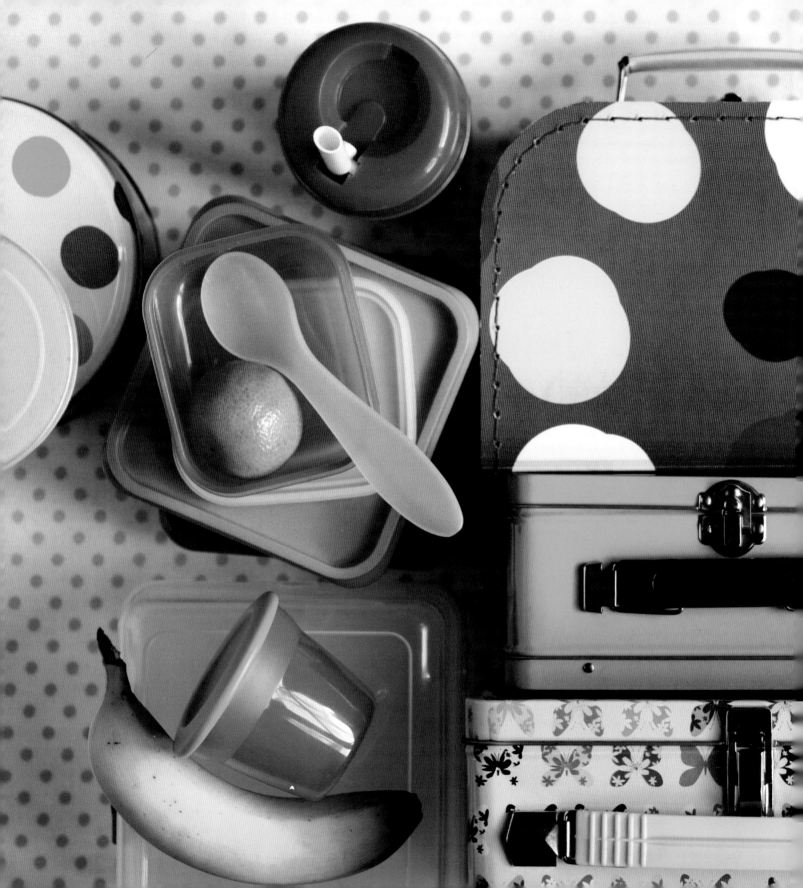

# packaging

### Keep it fresh

Some of the fresh food ideas in this book, like pâtés, cooked chicken, and yogurts, will need to be kept cool in the lunchbox. If you can, purchase an insulated lunchbox. Alternatively, add a small icepack to your child's lunchbox to help keep the contents fresh.

Similarly, any hot food will need to be kept hot, so it's good to invest in a good thermos. The small fat ones are best for children, because they can eat straight from them without having to decant the food into a bowl.

### Recycle

Once you start to make healthy lunchboxes for your child, you'll discover that you create less waste because you are no longer purchasing heavily packaged products.

When you make your child's packed lunch, try to keep the amount of packaging you use to a minimum and recycle anything left in the lunchbox. Involve your children by asking them to put their trash into the relevant trash cans, so that they get used to the idea of recycling. Remember trash in the trash can means more waste in the landfill site, and this is what we must avoid.

Try to avoid using plastic wrap, foil, plastic sandwich bags, and mixed packaging (e.g. drink cartons). These materials are not suitable for recycling (with the occasional exception of foil) and even though

the sandwich bags could be reused, they have a short lifetime and will end up in the trash sooner than a plastic tub.

### What should I use to store food in a lunchbox?

You should try to reuse things that you already have in your kitchen. You could even use an old ice cream container as a lunchbox.

### Small containers

Collect little airtight containers or cartons that dips, pasta sauces, or olives come in and keep them to store lunchbox snacks. You can also put yogurt into small cartons and wash them after using (just make sure the lid is airtight, so the yogurt doesn't leak out). If you buy individual yogurts, wash out the cartons and keep them so your children can use them for craft projects.

### Tin containers with plastic lids

Keep your eyes open for bargain containers, like metal ones with plastic lids that can be reused.

### Paper bags and greaseproof paper

Buy big packets of things, like biscuits, rather than buying them individually wrapped. Similarly, avoid packaged cheese slices. Instead, wrap up food like biscuits and cheese in paper bags or greaseproof paper.

### Ready-made packaging

Some food, especially items of fruit, like plums, apples, and oranges, come pre-packaged when they could easily

be sold loose. Try to buy fruit from your local market to avoid this unecessary packaging. If you are going to chop fruit into bite-size pieces, put them into small containers.

### Bottles

When you buy juice or water in small bottles, keep them so you can use them to store water and homemade smoothies. Try to avoid buying drinks in cartons because these are made from at least 3 materials—card, foil, and plastic—and cannot be recycled as the process is too expensive.

### Where your food comes from

Make your children aware of food miles by showing them on an atlas where their food has traveled from. The country of origin will usually appear on the packaging. Who has the packed lunch with the most food miles? Is it necessary to buy New Zealand apples when farmers grow them locally? Get your child to think about how they could have an altogether "greener" packed lunch?

### Fair trade

Many people in other countries work hard to produce the food we eat, yet they rarely get paid enough to feed their families. Next time you're in a supermarket, have a look at fair trade products like fresh fruit, yogurt, honey, sugar, and jam and think about why we should try to buy these wherever possible.

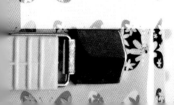

# menu planner

To help you on your way to producing healthy lunchboxes for your children, use this weekly menu planner as a starting point. As you prepare the lunches, think of how you can package them without creating excess waste.

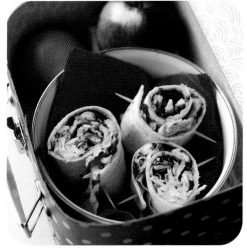

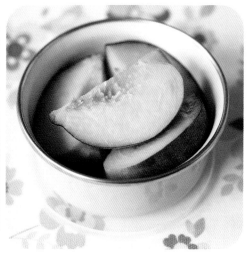

## monday

- turkey with cranberry sauce and lettuce wrap (see page 31)
- a handful of vegetable sticks
- a handful of dried fruits
- a piece of cheese and a cheese biscuit
- a drink of water

## tuesday

- tuna & sweetcorn pasta (see page 44)
- fresh peach—cut into quarters
- a fruity oat bar (see page 118)
- a drink of milk

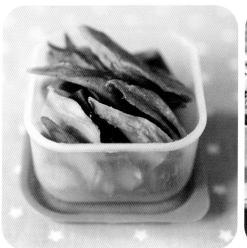

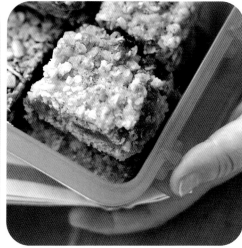

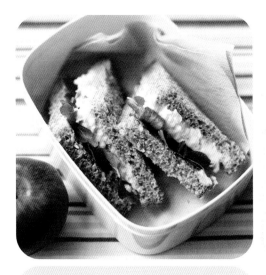

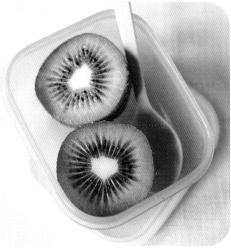

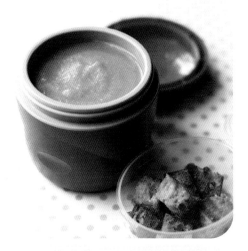

## wednesday

- egg salad & watercress sandwich (see page 32)
- a banana
- plain yogurt mixed with a little honey or fruit topping (see page 102)
- a drink of fruit juice

## thursday

- a sardine, lemon, and lettuce sandwich (see page 35)
- a handful of nuts and seeds
- a kiwi cut in half (with spoon for scooping out flesh)
- a smoothie (see page 99)

## friday

- butternut squash soup with Parmesan croutons (see page 61)
- yogurt with a little honey or fruit topping (see page 102)
- a satsuma
- 2 x muesli cookies (see page 118)
- a drink of water

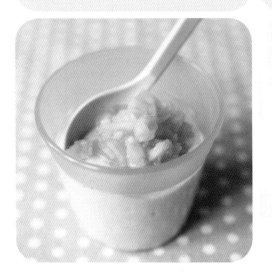

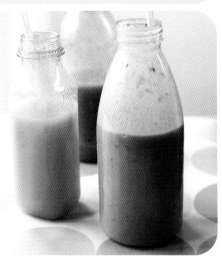

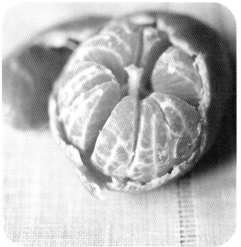

# index

## a

ADHD (attention deficit hyperactivity disorder) 34
almonds 9, 11
anxiety 34
apples 88
   apple and cheese sandwich 20
   apple puree 102
   green juice 99
   William's mini tarts 109
   yogurt toppings 102
apricots
   apricot and honey yogurt topping 102
   apricot slices 121
   cottage cheese and fruit sandwich 21
   fruity oat bars 118
asthma 11
avocados 11
   avocado and cream cheese sandwich 21
   avocado and hummus sandwich 23
   avocado and red bell pepper sandwich 24

## b

bacon
   puff pinwheels 78
   sandwiches 27, 32
   scones 85
bagels 18
balanced meals 6, 14
bananas 88, 99
   banana sandwiches 36
   yogurt topping 102
bean and sausage casserole 58
beef, horseradish, and cucumber sandwich 27
beet and cheese sandwich 20
   ham and beet pickle sandwich 28
   and hummus sandwich 23
bell peppers 69, 88
   avocado and red pepper sandwich 24
   chicken and red pepper stew 54
   cream cheese and red pepper sandwich 21
   egg, red pepper and cucumber sandwich 32
   sausage and red pepper rolls 69
betacarotene 69
biscuits
   cheese 91
   cheese and seed 96
   chocolate chip cookies 106
   cranberry 106
   fruity oat bars 118
   lemon shortbread with berries 105
   muesli cookies 118
blueberry muffins 108–9
bread 8, 14, 18
breadsticks 91
butternut squash soup 61

## c

cabbage, coleslaw 48
cakes
   apricot slices 121
   cereal bars 120
   chocolate cupcakes 117
   fruity oat bars 118
   golden raisin bake 103
   mini pear cakes 117
   muffins 108–9
   sticky gingerbread 114
calcium 10, 14, 81, 96, 113
carbohydrates 8, 14
carrots 88, 92
   bacon, watercress, and carrot sandwich 27
   carrot and hummus sandwich 23
   carrot, raisin, and peanut butter sandwich 36
   coleslaw 48
   pick 'n' mix salad 47
casserole, sausage, and bean 58
celery 88, 92
cereal bars 91, 120
cheese 9, 14, 91
   biscuits 91
   couscous with feta 40
   and cucumber sandwiches 36
   easy pizzas 70
   and ham sandwich 28
   and hummus sandwich 23
   mini quiches 74
   pesto cheese twists 66
   pick 'n' mix salad 47
   ploughman's sandwich 20
   popcorn 95
   puff pinwheels 78
   sandwiches 20–1
   scones 85
   and seed biscuits 96
   straws 66
chicken
   drumsticks 77
   and red bell pepper stew 54
   sandwiches 31
chickpeas 23
   chickpea dip 92
   falafel in pita 24
   hummus sandwiches 23
   sausage and bean casserole 58
chocolate
chocolate chip cookies 106
corn
   and tuna mini pasties 78
   and tuna pasta 44
   and tuna sandwich 35
cupcakes 117
chutney and sausage sandwich 28
ciabatta 18
coleslaw 48
constipation 8

cottage cheese
   and fruit sandwich 21
   and pineapple sandwich 21
couscous 40
cranberry cookies 106
cream cheese
   alfalfa 13
   dip 92
   sandwiches 20–1, 35
   egg and sprout sandwich 32
   salmon, tomato, and sprout sandwich 35
cucumber 88, 92
   beef, horseradish, and cucumber sandwich 27
   chicken, mango chutney, and cucumber sandwich 31
   couscous with 40
   and cream cheese sandwich 21
   egg, red bell pepper, and cucumber sandwich 32
   cheese and cucumber sandwich 36
   and peanut butter sandwich 36
   pick 'n' mix salad 47
   and tuna sandwich 35

## d

dehydration 12
depression 34
dips
   chickpea 92
   cream cheese 92
dried fruit 88
   carrot, raisin, and peanut butter sandwich 36
   chicken sandwich with fruit and nuts 31
   and cottage cheese sandwich 21
   fruit bread 18
   fruity oat bars 118
   golden raisin bake 103
   pick 'n' mix salad 47
   yogurt toppings 102
   drinks 12, 14
   juices 12
   smoothies 99

## e

eczema 11
eggs 6, 14
egg sandwiches 27, 32
   hard cooked 32
   mini quiches 74

## f

falafel in pita 24
fats 11
feta, couscous with 40
fiber 8, 23, 113
fish 6, 11, 14
mackerel *see* mackerel

oily 82
salmon *see* salmon
sandwiches 35
sardines *see* sardines
tuna *see* tuna
focaccia 18
French bread 18
fruit 9, 14, 88, 113
   fresh fruit jellos 110
   juice 12
   lemon shortbread with berries 105
   muffins 108–9
   pick 'n' mix salad 47
   smoothies 99
   yogurt toppings 102
   see also dried fruit
   fruit bread 18

## g

garlic 91
   pita crisps 91
gingerbread, sticky 114
grapes 88, 113
   pick 'n' mix salad 47
green juice smoothie 99

## h

ham
   easy pizzas 70
   sandwiches 28
   scones 85
herb scones 85
honey yogurt toppings 102
hummus 14, 92
   sandwiches 23
hydrogenated fats 11

## i

iron 77, 81

## j

jellos, fresh fruit 110

## k

kiwis 88, 99, 113

## l

lamb, mint jelly, and spinach sandwich 27
lemons
lemon jello 110
lemon shortbread with berries 105
lettuce
   bacon, lettuce, and tomato sandwich 27
   egg mayonnaise and lettuce sandwich 32
   green salad 51
   ham, tomato, and lettuce sandwich 28
   hummus, tomato, and lettuce

sandwich 23
sardines, lemon, and lettuce
   sandwich 35
tuna, cream cheese, and lettuce
   sandwich 35

**m**
mackerel 11
   smoked mackerel pâté 82
   smoked mackerel sandwich 35
magnesium 10
mangoes 99, 113
mayonnaise 32
meat 6, 11, 14
   roast meat sandwiches 27
menu planner 124–5
milk 11, 14, 91
   pink milk smoothie 99
minerals 10, 113
monounsaturated fats 91
muesli 102, 118

**n**
noodles 62
nuts 9, 11, 14, 91
   chicken sandwich with fruit and
      nuts 31
   nuts and seeds 91

**o**
oats 118, 120
olives 11
   easy pizzas 70
   Greek sandwiches 20
   scones 85
omega-3 fatty acids 11, 81, 82
onion and spinach tortilla 81
oranges 88, 99
orange jello 110
orange shortbread with berries 105

**p**
packaging 123
pasta 8, 14
   salads 44
pasties, tuna and sweetcorn 78
pastry
   cheese straws 66
   mini quiches 74
   pesto cheese twists 66
   puff pinwheels 78
   sausage and red bell pepper rolls 69
   tuna and corn pasties 78
   William's mini tarts 109
pâté, smoked mackerel 82
pea and salmon pasta 44
peanut butter sandwiches 36
peanuts 11
pears 88, 113
   mini pear cakes 117
pear and cream cheese sandwich 21

pesto
   cheese twists 66
   and cream cheese sandwich 21
   potato, pesto, and tuna salad 43
   puff pinwheels 78
   red pasta salad 44
pilchards 14
pineapple 62, 99, 113
   and cottage cheese sandwich 21
   noodles 62
pink milk smoothie 99
pita bread 18
   falafel in 24
   garlic pita crisps 91
pizzas, easy 70
ploughman's sandwich 20
polyunsaturated fats 91
popcorn 95
pork
   roast pork with apple sauce
      sandwich 27
   roast pork with chutney sandwich 27
potassium 81
potatoes 8
potato salads 43
processed foods 6, 10, 11
protein 7, 14
pulses 6, 23

**q**
quiches, mini 74

**r**
rainbow pot 88
raspberries 88, 99
raspberry jello 110
raspberry muffins 108–9
recycling 123
rice 8, 14
rice cakes 91
rolls 18

**s**
salads
   coleslaw 48
   couscous 40
   green 51
   pasta 44
   pick 'n' mix 47
   potato 43
salami, easy pizzas 70
salmon 11
   mini quiches 74
   and pea pasta 44
   sandwich 35
salt 10
sandwiches 17–36
   bacon 27, 32
   banana 36
   cheese 20–1
   chicken 31

egg 32
fish 35
Greek 20
ham 28
hummus 23
peanut butter 36
roast meats 27
salmon 35
sardine 35
sausage 28
shrimp 35
tuna 35
turkey 31
vegetarian 24
sardines 9, 11, 14
sardine sandwich 35
satsumas 113
saturated fats 11
sausages
   red pasta salad 44
   sausage and bean casserole 58
   sausage and red bell pepper rolls 69
   sausage sandwiches 28
sesame 73
   scones 85
   seeds 11
   cereal bars 120
   cheese and seed savory cookies 96
   nuts and seeds 91
semolina 40
sesame seeds
   hummus 92
   sausages 73
shortbread, lemon, with berries 105
shrimp sandwich 35
smoothies 99
snacks 73, 87–99
soup
   butternut squash 61
   tomato 57
soya milk and yogurt 9, 14
spinach 9
   and cream cheese sandwich 20
   green salad 51
   lamb, mint jelly, and spinach
      sandwich 27
   and onion tortilla 81
stew, chicken and red bell pepper 54
strawberries 99
   lemon shortbread with berries 105
   strawberry jello 110
stress 34
sugar 10
sunflower seeds 91

**t**
tofu 14
tomato 88
   bacon, egg, and tomato sandwiches
      27, 32

bacon, lettuce, and tomato sandwich
   27
cheddar, scallion, and tomato
   sandwich 20
cream cheese and sun-dried tomato
   sandwich 21
easy pizzas 70
ham, tomato, and lettuce sandwich
   28
hummus, tomato, and lettuce
   sandwich 23
and sausage sandwich 28
scones 85
soup 57
tuna, scallion, and tomato sandwich
   35
tortilla
   spinach and onion 81
   wraps 18
trans fats 11
tropical mix smoothie 99
tuna 11
   and corn mini pasties 78
   and corn pasta 44
   couscous with 40
   easy pizzas 70
   potato, pesto, and tuna salad 43
   sandwiches 35
turkey sandwiches 31

**v**
vegetables 14, 88, 113
   dips 92
   pick 'n' mix salad 47
vegetarian sandwiches 24
vitamin C 62, 69, 113
vitamin D 82

**w**
water 12
watercress
   bacon, watercress, and carrot
      sandwich 27
   egg mayonnaise and watercress
      sandwich 32
   green salad 51
   shrimp, mayonnaise and watercress
      sandwich 35
whole-grain foods 8
William's mini tarts 109

**y**
yogurt 9, 14, 91
   toppings 102

**z**
zinc 10, 31, 77

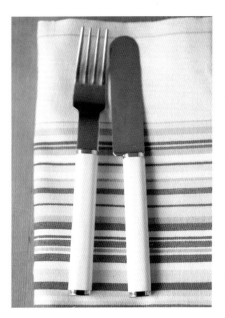

# acknowledgments

Thank you David for your love and trust, and to Ella, Lola, and Finley, my three biggest pickles in the pickle jar. Thanks Pop and Liz for being there. Mavis, I treasure our chats about food, recipes, and life. Thanks to Marcus and James for the fond memories and inspiration for the recipes.

Thanks to Vicki for helping create another exciting project, one that Lara and the Lara all-stars can enjoy.

Thanks to Alison, Iona, and Catherine and everyone involved in this book from Ryland Peters & Small.

Tara, I wished we lived closer, thanks for heading out of London so many times and for all the beautiful photos. Thanks to Chloe for your advice about rabbits and Liz for all the lunchboxes!

Brenda, thanks for your enthusiasm, help, and laughs, you look GOOD in a skirt and you are a great assistant!

Thanks to Annie from the Northmoor Trust, and the lovely Eka Morgan.

Well done to the models Ella, Lola & Finley; Sadie & Angus; Rory; Annabelle & Thomas; Violet; Ollie; Jemima; Liliana & Saskia; Biba; Erin; Hector; Matthew; Kitty; Ilaina & Huwaida. I hope you enjoy making and packing your own lunchboxes.

**Amanda Grant**

# conversion charts

Weights and measures have been rounded up or down slightly to make measuring easier.

Volume equivalents:

| American | Metric | Imperial |
|---|---|---|
| 1 teaspoon | 5 ml | |
| 1 tablespoon | 15 ml | |
| ¼ cup | 60 ml | 2 fl.oz. |
| ⅓ cup | 75 ml | 2½ fl.oz. |
| ½ cup | 125 ml | 4 fl.oz. |
| ⅔ cup | 150 ml | 5 fl.oz. (¼ pint) |
| ¾ cup | 175 ml | 6 fl.oz. |
| 1 cup | 250 ml | 8 fl.oz. |

1 stick butter = 8 tablespoons = 125 g

Weight equivalents:

| Imperial | Metric |
|---|---|
| 1 oz. | 25 g |
| 2 oz. | 50 g |
| 3 oz. | 75 g |
| 4 oz. | 125 g |
| 5 oz. | 150 g |
| 6 oz. | 175 g |
| 7 oz. | 200 g |
| 8 oz. (½ lb.) | 250 g |
| 9 oz. | 275 g |
| 10 oz. | 300 g |
| 11 oz. | 325 g |
| 12 oz. | 375 g |
| 13 oz. | 400 g |
| 14 oz. | 425 g |
| 15 oz. | 475 g |
| 16 oz. (1 lb.) | 500 g |
| 2 lb. | 1 kg |

Measurements:

| Inches | cm |
|---|---|
| ¼ inch | 5 mm |
| ½ inch | 1 cm |
| ¾ inch | 1.5 cm |
| 1 inch | 2.5 cm |
| 2 inches | 5 cm |
| 3 inches | 7 cm |
| 4 inches | 10 cm |
| 5 inches | 12 cm |
| 6 inches | 15 cm |
| 7 inches | 18 cm |
| 8 inches | 20 cm |
| 9 inches | 23 cm |
| 10 inches | 25 cm |
| 11 inches | 28 cm |
| 12 inches | 30 cm |

Oven temperatures:

| | | |
|---|---|---|
| 110°C | (225°F) | Gas ¼ |
| 120°C | (250°F) | Gas ½ |
| 140°C | (275°F) | Gas 1 |
| 150°C | (300°F) | Gas 2 |
| 160°C | (325°F) | Gas 3 |
| 180°C | (350°F) | Gas 4 |
| 190°C | (375°F) | Gas 5 |
| 200°C | (400°F) | Gas 6 |
| 220°C | (425°F) | Gas 7 |
| 230°C | (450°F) | Gas 8 |
| 240°C | (475°F) | Gas 9 |

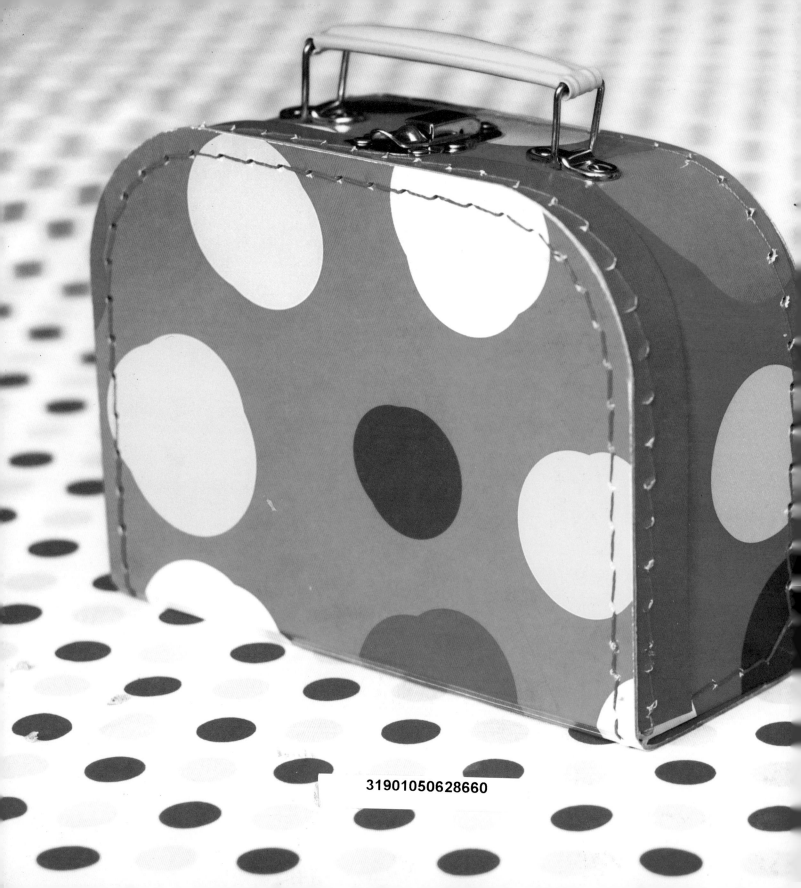

31901050628660